My **Dog** Has **Cancer.** What Can I Do?

*Nola's Wellness Guide & Journey
with Holistic Medicine*

HEATHER BEUKE DIERS

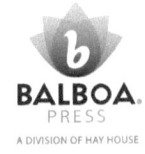

BALBOA
PRESS
A DIVISION OF HAY HOUSE

Balboa Press books may be ordered through booksellers or by contacting:

Balboa Press
A Division of Hay House
1663 Liberty Drive
Bloomington, IN 47403
www.balboapress.com
1 (877) 407-4847

Print information available on the last page.

ISBN: 978-1-5043-4964-2 (sc)
ISBN: 978-1-5043-4965-9 (e)

Balboa Press rev. date: 02/19/2016

Contributing Author: Heidi Straub - chapter, *Spiritual Healing & Meditation*.

Cover designed by Yu Zhang.

For Nola and Jean, the two most badass cancer warriors I've ever known. Because of you, my appreciation for clean food and holistic medicine has changed my life forever. I miss you both. xo

To all the other cancer warriors out there fighting with everything you have. Be informed and be empowered! I pray for every one of you.

Shout-outs

I want to give a special shout-out to all the people who helped when it really mattered. You supported me during Nola's journey with cancer and while writing, *My Dog Has Cancer. What Can I Do?*

Mark, thank you for loving our girl as much as I do. You made it possible for me to stay home to care for her, when she was sick, giving her a wonderful quality of life during a very scary time. You always support my decisions and make me laugh in dark moments. For that I am so grateful. I love you.

Dr. Cindy Baker, the best of both Eastern and Western medicine. Thank you for supporting our choice of holistic healthcare and for helping me create an amazing cancer fighting protocol for Nola. You always take great care of our pets and we are so lucky to have you in our area. Most of all, thank you for making Nola's last moments in this world so beautiful.

Juli, Anita and Ellen, thank you for letting me include you and your cancer warriors into our story. You were all an important part of our journey, along with so many others in the Artemisinin Yahoo Group. I will never be able to describe how much the support of this group has helped us along the way. We are forever bonded by this horrible disease, but at least something great came out of it...friendships.

Mark, Jen, Heidi, Susanne, Brian and Kerri, thank you for taking the time to read, edit and advise along the way. You each have your own amazing strengths in writing and journalism and I am so lucky to have had your insights, while editing, *My Dog Has Cancer. What Can I Do?*

Dawn, I'm so glad we took this publishing path together. Having a friend to share ideas and tips kept the journey exciting. You were a great motivator for me to keep writing and finish this book!

A special thank you to whoever reached out with a hug, Facebook message, text, email, gift, donation, card or phone call when Nola passed away. There are too many to list, which makes my heart swell every time I think of the outpouring of love that came to us at such a difficult time. It helped more than you will ever know.

Most importantly, thank you, God, for guiding me through every day of our cancer journey and through every page of this book. I am certain I would have never been able to get through any of it without You.

Disclaimer

Neither the author nor the publisher of this book is a veterinarian or other healthcare provider. This book documents the author's journey with her dog, Nola, canine cancer and everything she learned about holistic medicine, while treating Nola's cancer, Osteosarcoma.

This book is not intended to replace the care of a licensed veterinarian or other healthcare provider and is not intended to diagnose or treat any disease without a licensed veterinarian or other healthcare provider's guidance.

The author, publisher and all other contributors will not be liable for any damages in connection with the use of this book. This book is the opinion of the author, with regard to treating cancer holistically. It is a resource meant to aid the immune system and enhance the quality of life of a canine cancer patient, while under the care of a licensed veterinarian or other healthcare provider.

You should always consult your veterinarian and other healthcare providers before giving any food, vitamins, supplements or other treatments to your pets.

Introduction
My Mission

The intent of this book is not to persuade you to do exactly as we did; rather, it is meant to inform you of many cancer fighting remedies that fall outside of Western medicine. Telling our story is a way to create something good and helpful out of a horrible disease.

This book provides you with important information that will guide you through every stage, while you make difficult decisions regarding the care of your cancer warrior dog. Writing this journal was also my therapy and a forum to remember our journey together with our girl, Nola. I want to give her life meaning, as well as her illness. Because of her illness, I took a crash course in cancer treatments, mostly natural, and learned more in two years about nutrition than most doctors learn in a lifetime.

After completing hundreds of hours of research and taking a great team of veterinarians' advice, I have created an economical, cancer-fighting and immune-building protocol for any animal (or human!) fighting cancer.

The problem we had was time. It took many months of intense research to develop our protocol, during a crucial time in my baby girl's life. **My mission is to save you time on research and give you an advantage over this evil we call cancer.**

Nola had <u>Osteosarcoma</u> (OS), which is an incurable, fast spreading bone cancer that would not wait while I tried to catch up on my research. As Nola's mommy and caregiver, I felt her life was in my hands. Nola always came to me for protection and she knew I had her back, no matter what. Ironically, I was already researching natural cancer cures because I had a friend, Jean, who was fighting cancer with many natural remedies. I was fascinated by the idea *food is medicine.* I had learned a lot from Jean about the importance of nutrition when fighting a disease. Whole foods, herbs & spices should never be discounted as a secondary option for healthcare - a healthy diet *is* the foundation of a successful battle.

The desire to learn more about food's medicinal properties lead to a few vegan cooking classes, which were invaluable during this process. I feel my jumpstart on proper nutrition helped to slow Nola's cancer early on, buying precious time with our girl, while I continued my research.

We were able to turn her first diagnosis of "three-months-to-live" into a year of a great quality of life. These, by the way, are the same results that many OS dogs get with early amputation and chemotherapy. Her cancer was not curable, so our goal was to keep her body healthy and strong, for as long as possible, by creating an environment in which cancer could not thrive. I also feel certain we could have turned that year into more time if we had started with the protocol with which we ended.

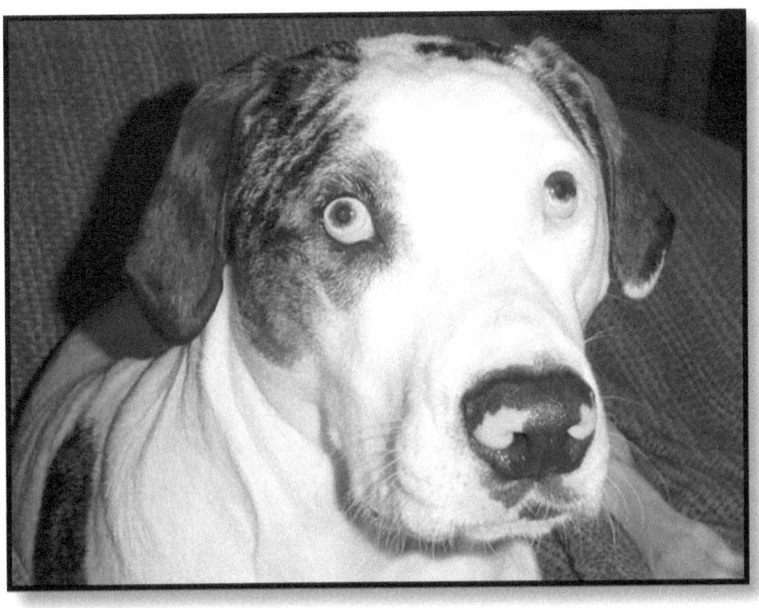

Any extra time we are given with our loved ones is a gift and I want that for every family that is fighting this evil disease.

I pray you can benefit from all that my journey with Nola has taught me. From the mistakes we made, to the resources that guided and supported us. Our strategy ultimately extended and improved the quality of Nola's last year of life and it can do the same for your warrior. May you find what you need, within the pages of this book, to extend your journey with your cancer warrior and make it a beautiful one.

Nola's Journey Includes:

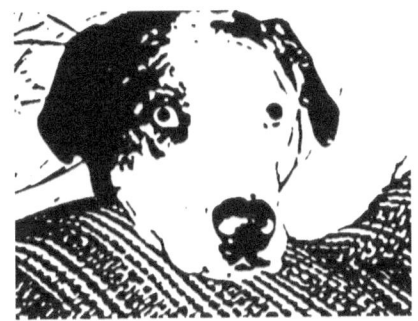

My dog has cancer.

What can I do?

Let me begin by expressing my deepest sympathy for the devastating news that your beloved has cancer. I still remember the feeling I had when I stood in disbelief after finding out our precious Nola had <u>Osteosarcoma</u> (OS). I felt as if my soul had left my body and I was standing outside the room watching someone else's life. The thoughts were racing through my mind, "But it was just a *slight* limp, in fact we weren't even sure she *was* limping and she looks so healthy. We cook all of her meals and we don't feed her crappy dog treats, how can this be?" Then, as our veterinarian (at the time) started rattling on about how Nola only had three months to live, I remember drifting off again thinking, "What can I do to help my girl?" Being somewhat of a control freak and too stubborn to give into this evil disease and arbitrary statistics, I knew my girl wasn't going to die in three months – not if I had anything to do about it.

After he gave me the information for our next meeting with the surgeon, explaining how surgery and chemotherapy were our only options, I knew he would not be a part of our journey for long. I said, "Thank you very much," left his office and immediately went into research mode. I spent the next eight months cramming for what felt like the most important exam I have ever taken; my baby girl's life depended on whether I passed or failed. I knew our funds were limited and our veterinarian did not believe in holistic medicine and cancer fighting diets, which explains why his patients were only living for three months with this type of cancer. I knew he would be of no help to me long term and time was of the essence.

I had to act fast, pull my team together and make the right decisions quickly, while not second guessing myself. Well, that last part is almost impossible because I constantly had to second guess everything in order to keep an open mind and maintain a sense of reality. I didn't want to convince myself of something that wasn't possible, but I also didn't want to be blinded by statistics from a veterinarian who didn't understand the importance of nutrition over chemo, radiation or surgeries. It all has to work together and if the diet does *not* come first, none of the other treatments will have the outcome for which you are hoping.

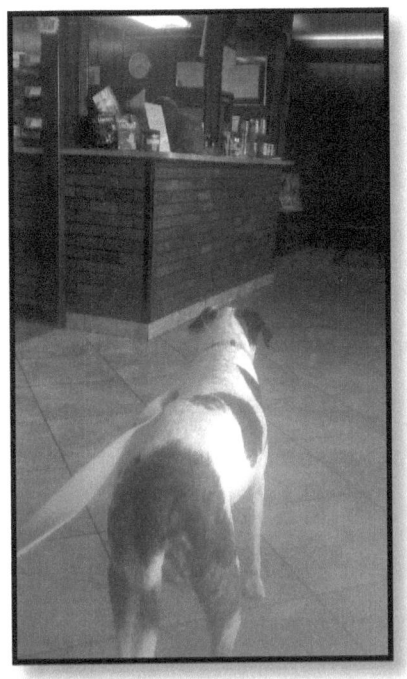

This picture captures the very last "normal" moment before our lives changed forever. This is Nola staring down the veterinarian's cat on the counter, right before we went back to find out Nola's lump on her leg was Osteosarcoma and we were getting ready to go to war with cancer.

As you can see, I knew immediately I was 'all in' to help my girl fight, no matter how long or how hard. As long as she was up for it, so was I. The first question I want you to ask yourself is, "are you in for whatever it takes?" You need to come by this question honestly, because the experience can be daunting at times - draining both physically and financially.

Even if you choose the holistic route, you still have a lot of vet bills and supplements, which all add up. The time required for care is 24/7 – you are basically providing your warrior around the clock hospice care. It doesn't mean you can't work or leave the house, but you are always on call. Of course, if you are anything like we are, the answer is simple because none of that matters. There was nothing we wouldn't do for our girl and giving up on her was never on the table. All that mattered was keeping her healthy, comfortable and most of all happy, for as long as possible, with the means we had available. I'm telling you this to prepare you, not to scare you. I have no doubt if we can do it, anyone can. All you can give is your best – no more, no less. You get through it one day at a time. I am not promising you a healthy diet that follows our protocol will cure your dog's cancer. I will promise you, without a strong cancer fighting diet & protocol, you will most likely not win the battle long term. I have watched many cancer dogs fight successfully for several years on nothing more than a strong cancer fighting diet and holistic medicine. I have also watched many dogs fight with equal success by utilizing surgery, chemotherapy and radiation; however, they all combine them with a healthy, cancer fighting diet as the foundation of their treatment to ensure their pets' immune systems remain strong as their bodies are hit with the harsh elements of the procedures.

My goal for this book is to make this journey less daunting for you. I want to save you time in research and provide you with a tool to get started fighting cancer immediately. That doesn't mean you won't have your own homework and research, but I invite you to start here and follow the links I have provided to help you further your search in the right direction. What to do first? Before you do anything else, including finishing this book, I think you should take a minute to join the Yahoo support groups I mention in the next chapter, which is a great way to start building your team.

The next step to building your team is to find a veterinarian who practices holistic medicine and/or Traditional Chinese Medicine (TCM) to fight cancer. It may be necessary to have two veterinarians, one western medicine and one holistic. If you have more than one, make sure you are up front with both, from the beginning, that they are a part of a team and they are to share your warrior's medical records with each other at all times. For this reason, it is best to find one who does both, but it's not always possible, depending on where you live and who is available.

Several people in the Artemisinin Yahoo Group recommend Dr Charles Loops, who is a well known homeopathic veterinarian who offers phone consultations and provides information on his website. He is a good option, if you don't have a holistic vet near you, but I would seek out a local holistic veterinarian as your first choice. I feel it is important for them to work with you and your dog in person.

We were blessed to have Dr. Cindy Baker, who is the perfect blend of east meets west, looking after our girl. Her practice is Bargersville Veterinary Hospital and Wellness Center in Bargersville, Indiana. There was a period of time when we were transitioning from our original vet, who first diagnosed Nola, to Dr. Baker and I made sure they were both completely informed at all times, which is how Nola's journal originated.

Both vets should be willing to work with you on a protocol that includes a healthy cancer fighting diet, holistic medicine and the best options for chemotherapy and radiation, if you decide on that path. You will find a lot of support for all options in the yahoo groups, so feel free to ask questions to the groups about their experiences, as you proceed and are faced with major decisions. I have included as much information as I can about our experiences and comprehensive protocol that took us months to develop, hoping you will have even more success than we did by starting it sooner.

Your team will also include an oncologist, especially if you plan to use chemotherapy as part of your protocol. And you may need a surgeon, depending on the type of cancer you are fighting. We never saw an oncologist throughout our entire journey, which was not completely intentional and not necessarily my recommendation to you, but it ended up working out fine for us. Especially, since we opted to remain 100% holistic with regard to cancer fighting medications.

After Nola's diagnosis, we immediately met with our surgeon, which by coincidence was the same surgeon who performed Nola's ACL surgeries on her rear knees when she was two years old. He had done a fantastic job and knowing he was looking after Nola again put us at ease. We have since learned he is known in our area as a brilliant and highly respected surgeon, which *we* already knew, but it was nice to have it validated. I left our first appointment feeling very clear headed and focused because he helped us make a couple fast decisions for the best plan for Nola's fight and we never looked back.

After our first appointment we had a plan, which was more than I could have hoped for at that point. Surprisingly, he talked us out of the meeting with the oncologist. He knew money was not in excess for us and we had to be careful where we chose to spend it. He explained that we could set up the meeting with the oncologist to run tests to confirm the diagnosis, but he had no doubt it was OS after looking at Nola's x-rays. We were told the same by our vet, so we decided a $1000 test to tell us what we already knew was not where we should spend our money at that moment. We needed to put that money toward a custom boot to protect her tumor leg from unnecessary damage. I talk more about this boot in the chapter, *Is Amputation Right For Us?*

He briefly mentioned he was not a fan of chemotherapy and he didn't go into great detail as to why. Probably because I didn't ask, since I too was not a fan of chemotherapy and I understood the theory. I was not convinced it was going to help any more than natural remedies, since Nola's cancer was not curable, and it could possibly harm her. Holistic medicine was the road I was more comfortable traveling. I have since learned a little more about canine chemotherapy and how it compares to human chemotherapy. My view on canine chemo is not quite as negative as it was before, because I learned that some types of canine chemotherapy is not as damaging to healthy cells as human chemotherapy. Since I did not focus my energy researching it further, I can't go into any more detail on the topic, but this is a great conversation for you to have with your veterinarian. I still remain hesitant to recommend it because I have seen some dogs die very quickly after treatments. I am convinced it depends on the strength of your dog's immune system before treatment, which falls back on proper nutrition.

In addition to the Yahoo cancer groups, veterinarian (both holistic and western medicine), oncologist and surgeon (if needed), you need your home team in place. Your family and friends will help you stay sane as well as help with some of the responsibility, especially if you work outside the home and need to administer meds while you are away. Sometimes you just need to vent and cry or, better yet, you need to surround yourself with people who will give you the release of a good laugh. We all know laughter is the very best kind of medicine. Most importantly, you need to know who in your household is the primary caregiver. You should communicate with each other frequently on medicine doses, feeding times, etc. I recommend a food & supplement chart to help with tracking your doses. I have shared our chart in the appendix, but you should revise it to work with your protocol and schedule. Plus, mine made sense to me, but my husband (who is very intelligent) could never figure it out, so you may not either.

You will be frustrated and sad at times because you are human and it is completely natural. Just remember your pets can hear you and they know when you are upset, which hinders their ability to heal. It is important to create a healing environment of peace and love and to remember your pets are living in the moment - you will hear this a lot because it's true. They don't know they have cancer and they aren't worried about the past or their future, as they only care about the now. Focus on making the now as fun and comfortable for them as possible, which is all that really matters in the end.

Our favorite way to enjoy the 'now' was by taking family road trips. Nola and Barley both loved car rides, so we took them out as much as possible. Sometimes we would go to the park and other times we would just drive around with no real destination in mind. Look at those smiles and tell me they weren't having the time of their lives. I know I was.

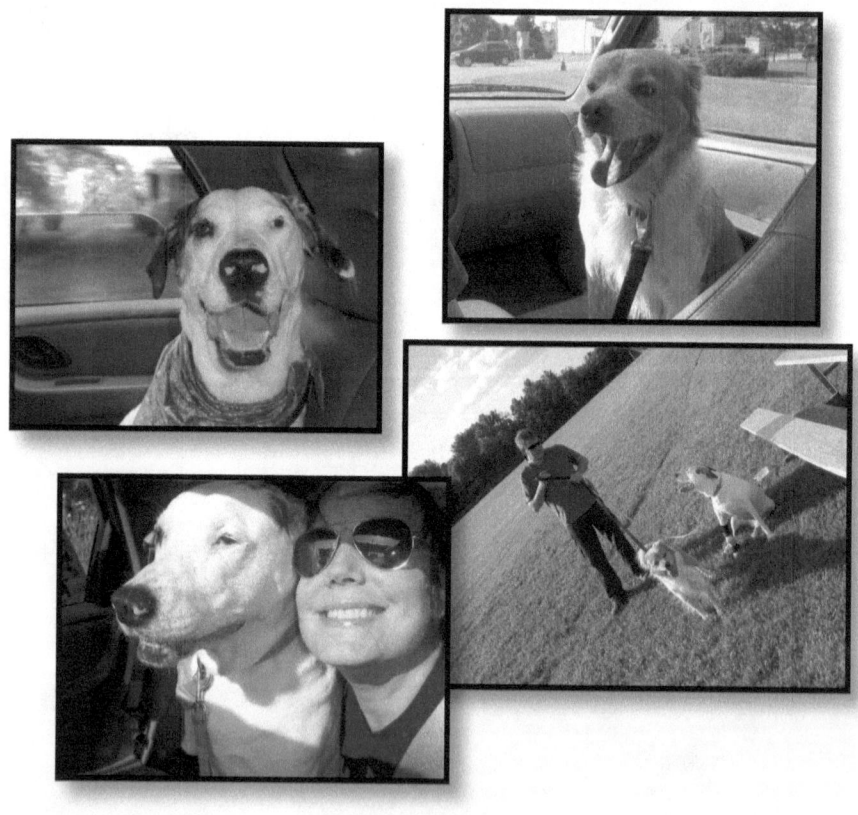

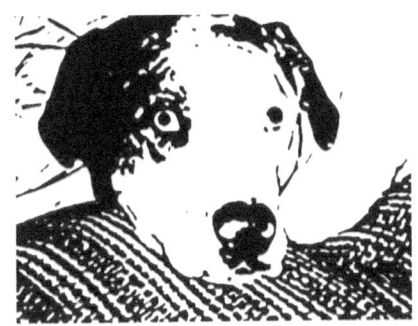

Support Groups

~ It takes a village

You will gain more knowledge and support within these groups than you will from any one veterinarian. There are people from all over the world in the groups, connecting and answering each others' questions. They share information from their veterinarians and home remedies with which they have had success. I'm not suggesting that our veterinarians are lacking in any way, but there is no way one person can learn everything there is to know about any one disease. This is why it makes sense to converse with people all over the world who are gleaning information from their veterinarians and sharing all of their best advice. Questions are responded to very quickly and at all hours of the night; it seems as though someone is always awake and ready to help. Everyone in these groups knows exactly what you are going through and they bring so much love and encouragement, which becomes invaluable while making it through this journey. I am still learning new things from them that I apply to my healthy dogs for prevention. Although I've never met any of them in person, I feel like we are friends for life bound by this horrible disease. I have no doubt you will have the same experience, so I am suggesting that joining the groups should be your **very first step in this journey**.

I think you should join all three groups I mention, but if you choose only one, my favorite is the <u>Artemisinin Yahoo Group</u>, of which I am still a member. The people in this group are great sources of strength and empowerment and their resources seem to be endless. I like to stay current on any new information they share about the latest cancer treatments from around the world. Not to mention, <u>Artemisinin</u> appears to be a huge factor in the success of many of the cancer dogs I have been following, whether they are 100% holistic or combine holistic medicine with chemotherapy. <u>Artemisinin</u> is more or less nature's chemotherapy and has proven to work with many forms of cancer. When you join this group, you will learn everything there is to know

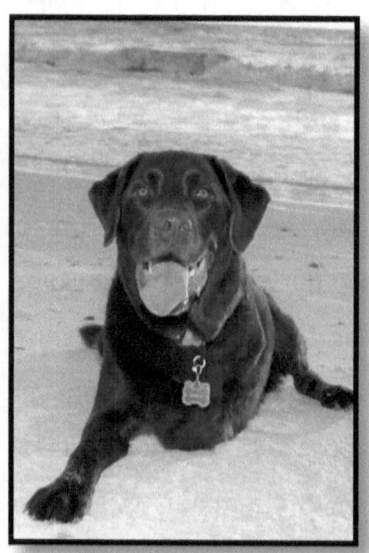

about Artemisinin, but keep in mind that you can be in the group whether or not you choose to use Artemisinin.

Ellen Venturella-Wilson is one of the moderators of the group and the proud mom of Charley (shown here), who was an OS survivor for over 4 years! Charley continues to be our inspiration, even though he earned his angel wings and crossed the bridge June 2, 2015. Knowing he was able to survive OS for over 4 years gives us all hope, because we know it is possible. Those statistics are typically unheard of with Osteosarcoma and she contributes a lot of Charley's success to Artemisinin. Charley did take chemotherapy after two different surgeries and he is one of the reasons I am now on the fence regarding canine chemotherapy. However, I am confident the chemo would not have saved him from OS for so long, if Charley had not also been taking Artemisinin and eating a cancer fighting diet. Not all dogs respond to Artemisinin the same way, but Charley is definitely a poster child for this natural cancer killer and a constant reminder to never give up hope. Ellen shares her protocol for Charley in the archives, so once you join the group, you will have access to her information as well.

Artemisinin and Cancer – "This is a group for people who are using Artemisinin and/or its analogs to treat their dog's cancer or who are interested in networking with others who are using these experimental compounds. Since research with Artemisinin and cancer is still in its infancy and much of what is known about the success of ART compounds with cancer is anecdotal, I wanted to provide a forum for people to share their experiences using this promising new herbal extract. This is not a group which offers medical advice; it is to share anecdotal information and experience with Artemisinin and cancer."

http://pets.groups.yahoo.com/group/artemisinin_and_cancer/

Bone Cancer Dogs – "In memory of Marcie…..Our group is dedicated to dogs with Osteosarcoma & other bone cancers and to their guardians who fight bravely. It is a place for support, comfort, guidance, learning, hope and encouragement. It was inspired by Rowdy Roddy Piper, a Rottweiler who lost his fight to bone cancer on September 2, 2004."
http://pets.groups.yahoo.com/group/bonecancerdogs/

Tripawds – "Tripawds is your three legged dog resource and help center. This is a community of support for sharing your story and learning from others about amputation for dogs, canine Osteosarcoma or other cancers, and loving life on three legs."
http://tripawds.com/

The Tripawds Group is a fabulous group to join if you do decide amputation surgery is going to be part of your journey. They will help you with every issue that comes up, both pre-surgery and post surgery, and they will help you to realize most dogs get around absolutely fine on three legs. It is invaluable to have a forum that answers all the questions you have, to help your dog easily transition from four legs to three and to thrive as a new member of the Tripawd society.

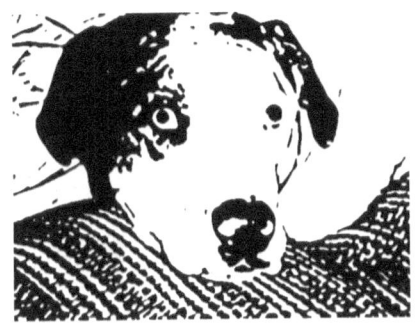

Getting to know Nola

~ Our Little Badass

When I try to describe Nola in one word, it always comes down to badass. Don't get me wrong, she was a very friendly dog who never met a stranger. She was a social butterfly from day one and commanded the attention of everyone in the room, until her very last days. She was afraid of nothing and she had a gift of communication - demanding what she wanted, including respect, and getting it. If you met her, you either loved her or hated her, but you NEVER ignored her. She was mostly loved because, even when she was pushy and demanding, she was so brilliant and clever about it that you couldn't help admiring her. From the time she was a small puppy to later as a senior dog, her life was a continuous game of how to outsmart the humans and she had mastered it.

I will never forget the first time she tricked me, when she was a pretty young dog, into getting up from the chair we were sharing. She decided she wanted it all to herself, so she made several attempts to push me off. I told her *she* would have to move, because I was still watching TV and I didn't want to get up yet. So, she got up, went over to the door and asked to go outside. Not thinking much about it, I got up and went to the door to let her

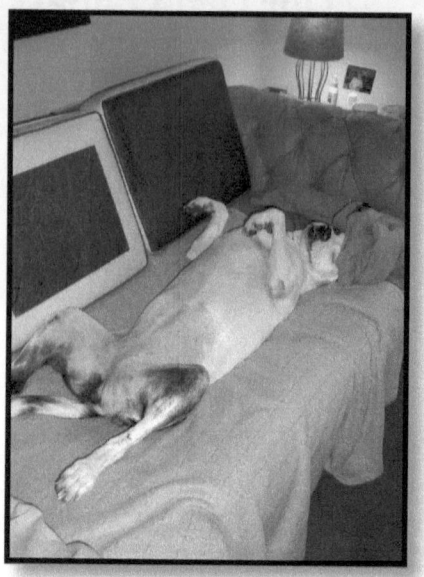

out just as she ran past me, jumped back into the chair and stretched out, while letting out a huge sigh as if to say, "sucker." She did this to me many more times over the years and I always seemed to fall for it. If we ever let down our guard, she was there to seize the moment. This is a picture of her stealing my spot

on the couch when I got up for a cup of coffee. Can you see her evil little grin? I can. She loved to tease her mommy and she was rotten. She was perfect in every way.

By the time she was a senior – she lived to be almost twelve – she pretty much ran our household. She determined when we ate, slept, went out, stayed home...everything revolved around her wants and needs. The truth be told, we loved every minute of it.

She was the greatest dog as an adult because she was wicked smart, fearless, strong (even when she was ill), loving and silly.

She *was* extremely bossy, however, and as she matured, her bossy nature grew from a bratty, mischievous youngster to our elder in the home who demanded her way and accepted nothing less. She made it pretty clear she had no patience for the word "no" and she had no problem letting us know when we fell short of her expectations. "Just give her what she wants, it's easier that way," was the unspoken (and sometimes spoken) word in our home, after years of training she had instilled in us. She was relentless in her determination and would wear us down no matter how long it took to get her way. Over time we decided it was much easier to just obey her. Anyone who owns a Catahoula knows the determination I am talking about. They simply never give up.

Of course, I say these things in a joking manner (sort of) because she was not as bad as I am describing. She was so silly, had a witty sense of humor and she loved to tease us. She especially loved to get a rise out of me, looking at me with a big smile on her face and wagging her tail when I raised my voice in frustration. I have never met a dog who actually enjoyed getting reprimanded, until I met Nola. She would do anything for attention, even if it was negative attention, and she had my number from day one. She knew I loved her devious little mind. She earned my respect by marching to the beat of her own drum. She knew right from wrong, but it had to be on her terms – I can relate, I'm the exact same way.

Once Nola was diagnosed with cancer our respect for her grew even stronger. Through her fight, she taught us so much about strength and endurance, which is how the nickname Badass came to be. It did not come from her bossy & stubborn nature, although I do know her stubborn attitude helped her a lot in her fight with cancer. I call her Badass because she showed us over and over it was possible to keep fighting every single day without ever feeling sorry for herself.

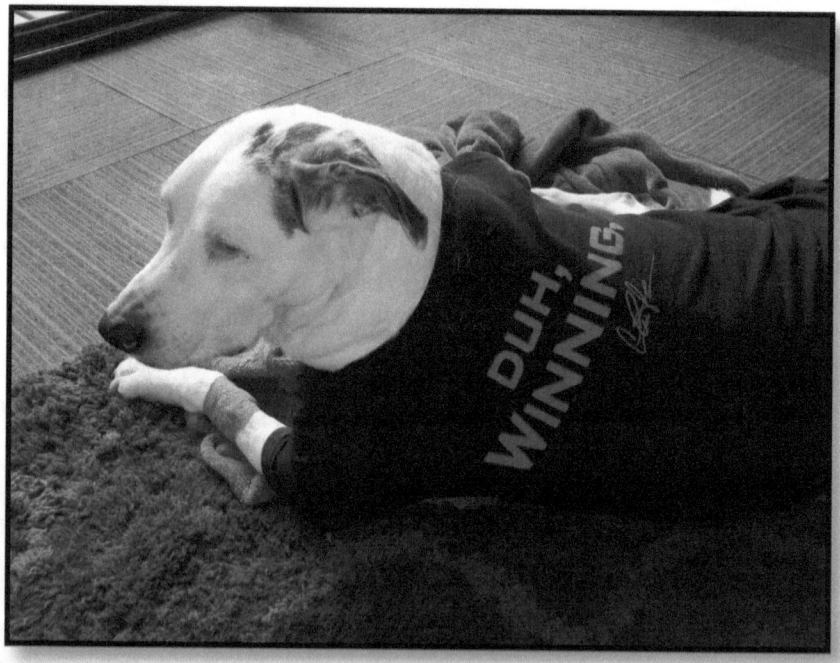

She never gave into pain and she never let her illness slow her down. Again, she was too damn stubborn to give into it. And for such a stubborn old girl, she was the best patient in the world.

She would let us feed her anything, while showing us complete trust. I truly believe she understood that everything we gave her was to help her. This was the same dog I would typically have to chase around the house to give a pill, in the past. She knew what I gave her made her feel better; therefore, she let us continue to give her everything necessary to keep her comfortable. She took pills like a champ, she let us give her apple cider vinegar water and lemon water at all hours of the day and she ate every concoction of food we could dream up and never turned her nose. She was so brave. Her will to live and bravery made her fight very manageable, sometimes even enjoyable and always inspirational.

We learned to live in the moment – remember I mentioned this is something you will hear a lot from many people along this journey. In my opinion, it is the most important lesson you will learn from this experience and will hopefully carry on with your future pets. If you can keep each moment as happy as possible, which includes keeping pain managed and its body strong, you are succeeding in this fight. Don't get caught up in trying to predict its future - this was a hard lesson for me to learn. With every triumph, it became more apparent that it was ALL about the triumphs and very little about the potential of the evil disease.

As brilliant as Nola was, she still did not know that she had cancer and she didn't really care to know as long as she was getting her way and ruling our household. I would love to go on forever about her tenacity, like how she drug me down our road (on three legs at this point) when she was at her sickest and insisted on going on a walk. No matter how weak she was and how many breaks she had to take along the way, she was going on that walk, damn it! She was too heavy for me to carry and too damn stubborn to turn around, so I had no choice but to stand by her side, while she pushed and fought harder to get down that road than I have fought for anything in my life – other than fighting her cancer, of course.

I could tell you stories like this for the remainder of the book, but you have a fight of your own for which to prepare and a lot of important information you need to digest in a timely manner. You will have your own stories about your own journey with your little badass cancer warrior and I pray you find the following information clear, concise and helpful in your fight. My goal is to inspire you and convince you that you DO have options and you do not have to pay attention to statistics, because every dog is different.

I encourage you to question EVERYTHING your veterinarian and oncologist suggest. I don't want you to question with doubt, because I hope you have chosen a team of doctors you trust completely. Ask questions so you fully understand what every drug is meant to accomplish and whether or not it has side effects that might make its journey less than a pleasant one. Remember, at the end of the day, you have the final say in its care and knowledge is the only way to make an educated decision about your choices – knowledge is power.

Knowledge was at the core of our journey, which became a journey of health and happiness and I let Nola drive the bus – like I had a choice. Nola's life was always about being in control of the wheel and her fight against cancer was no different. As I said before, I could go on forever about our girl, but you have work to do. However, if you want to get to know Nola a little better and read about her experiences along the way, feel free to become her friend on Facebook, where we continue to keep her badass spirit alive. During our fight, we used her Facebook page to document her journey, so hopefully you will glean some additional support and motivation from her day to day experiences.

https://www.facebook.com/nola.diers

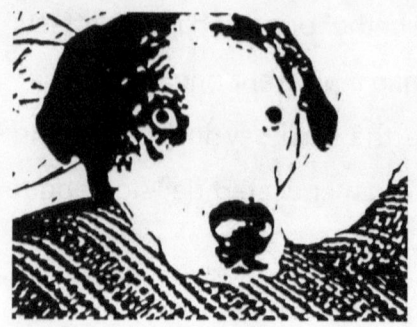

Nutrition ~ Mother Nature provides the best medicine

When fighting cancer, there are a few universal rules that anyone who does the most basic research can learn; however, your doctors (both for humans and for animals) rarely know this information or give it the value it deserves. I am completely perplexed by how little nutrition is taught or utilized in Western medicine for the treatment of cancer or any other disease.

The year prior to Nola's diagnosis, her body sent us many signals we overlooked and misunderstood. I now know they were symptoms of an auto-immune condition and we made the mistake of treating the symptoms instead of the cause. Nola continuously had a severe rash on her belly, her skin was dry and flaky and her coat was thin and brittle. Her vet at the time (not Dr. Cindy Baker) was treating her for allergies, alternating antibiotics, Benadryl and steroids. All of which were detrimental to her immune system, making the symptoms worse over time. Pair that with her last round of vaccination shots that she should have never received, as a ten year old dog with a compromised immune system, and you have the perfect recipe for cancer, which she was diagnosed with a few months later.

I was able to determine later that her issues were auto-immune related, not allergies, because all her symptoms went away once I began enhancing her food with these wonderful nutrients. Her rash disappeared, her skin was no longer flaky & her coat turned very thick and shiny – this was AFTER a cancer diagnosis. It was that simple.

When I look back at her symptoms, I feel ignorant and embarrassed for not realizing she was basically malnourished – it is so obvious to me now. We had always cooked Nola's food from scratch because she also had food allergies, which were diagnosed when she was younger. I am the first to admit, we had gotten lazy with her food preparation over the years. We simplified the process with a stew of ground turkey and frozen vegetables, which worked well for her as a younger dog, but we did not provide her with all the additional nutrients needed as she aged into a senior dog. I was also not aware at the time that dogs need their vegetables to be pureed, before feeding them, because their bodies don't break down vegetables the way humans do. Pureeing them will ensure its body gleans their nutrients before they pass through your dog's short digestive tract. I promise you, I will never make these mistakes again. Watching her rash clear up so fast with healthy food, herbs & spices, when we struggled for years using Big Pharma, was eye opening and a great lesson of the power of food.

How you treat the body will affect the outcome – this thought should empower you!

I am getting ready to blow your mind further by simplifying how cancer works in the body and explaining how to create a cancer killing environment with, wait for it...FOOD! The following is true for both humans and canines, because cancer is cancer. Cancer thrives in an acidic environment and it feeds off sugar. Conversely, omega-3 starves cancer, by oxygenating the blood. **Cancer cannot thrive or survive in an oxygenated, alkaline environment**.

This information is a game-changer in your fight and knowledge is your secret weapon to controlling the disease. To be clear, I'm not claiming this is the next miracle cure for cancer and it's the answer to everything, but it *is* basic chemistry that can't be disputed. There is scientific evidence proving cancer can't survive in an oxygenated, alkaline environment, so doesn't it make sense to do everything possible to create an oxygenated, alkaline environment in your warrior's body? I think so and I promise it won't make things worse. This is a link to an article by Dr. Otto Warburg that shares results from his many years of research on the topic, http://cancercompassalternateroute.com/cancer-5/ cancer-cannot-survive-in-an-oxygenated-alkaline-environment/.

The first step in your protocol is to **cut out all sugars**, including grains and simple carbohydrates, which turn to sugar in the body. This means **no more kibble dog food**. Many people cut out all fruit as well with the theory sugar is sugar, but I disagree with this theory. Yes, you should be careful with the quantity of fruit intake, but Mother Nature knows her stuff. She packs so many antioxidants into a blueberry it only takes a very small amount to have a huge impact on the immune system. The benefits far outweigh the very small amount of sugar obtained. Many fruits are also alkalizing, so choose your fruit wisely and stay away from fruit high in sugar with little antioxidant or alkalizing properties. I include the ones I believe to be safe and beneficial in the following list.

The second step is **oxygenating the blood** with very high levels of omega-3 fatty acids. For dogs, fish oil pills are the easiest way to accomplish this, because you can open them and pour them directly onto its food. This is easier than feeding the pills whole and dogs typically love the fishy smell and taste. I will talk about dosing quantities in the next chapter, *Vitamins & Supplements*.

Along with fish oil pills, add food high in omega-3 like salmon, tuna, flax (flax oil & ground flax seeds), wheatgrass and spirulina.

Although chia seeds are an excellent source of omega-3 fatty acids for humans, I wouldn't rely on them for an omega-3 source for your cancer dog. They won't hurt it, but as I mentioned before, it's hard for dogs to break down and absorb omega-3 from plant sources that haven't been pureed or ground. I would save your chia seeds for your salads and smoothies; don't waste them in your canine warrior's food. Wheatgrass and spirulina are plant sources, but you typically use them in powder form or as fresh juice, which are completely broken down. Its body doesn't have to do much work to absorb the nutrients. Chia seeds take longer to break down; therefore, they pass through the short digestive tract before it has the chance to absorb them. Flax seeds, which are also very high in Omega-3, are a better option than chia seeds, since they are to be ground before eaten. Flax oil is an even better option for your canine, for the same reasons I mentioned before, it is absorbed into the body faster.

The third step is to pack every meal with **alkaline and anti-inflammatory foods**, which I include in this chapter.

To recap, **no sugar + high doses of omega-3 fatty acids + alkaline foods = an environment in which cancer can't thrive**. Very simple. This information is easy to find on the internet. The Gerson Institute has been healing patients with cancer and other diseases, with this same method, for years. Kris Carr, the Crazy

Sexy Cancer chic, has been beating all odds for over a decade while fighting a rare and incurable stage 4 cancer with a plant base, holistic lifestyle. She has many books on the topic and a great blog – look her up!

The information is easily attainable, yet our mainstream healthcare providers either don't know this information or they simply don't find it important enough to apply to their main healthcare protocol. This isn't practical when you think about it, because it is basic science!

Everyone's body has had potential cancer cells running through it at any given time, this we know. Our bodies, when healthy and toxin free, are designed to kill and discard the abnormal cells, before they attach themselves and multiply, which is how cancer begins. We are equipped to take care of it ourselves, when properly nourished.

Since science proves that keeping our bodies nourished with whole food *is* the foundation of good health, I believe this is why we have more cancer now than ever before. Our society lives off processed foods - no one seems to cook meals from scratch anymore. We have decided fast food is a sufficient dinner to feed our families and the same is true for our pets. We tend to buy large economy bags of pet food with cheap, unhealthy additives and we wonder why canine and feline cancer is so common. Don't get me started on GMO labeling – that is a discussion for another book, but it is relevant to this epidemic.

Following is my list of foods I alternated for Nola's cancer fighting meals. I am not suggesting everything on this list goes into every meal. I believe alternating is better for fighting cancer, so the body doesn't get used to any one nutrient and learn to compensate for it. Cancer is very smart and it learns ways to camouflage itself in the body. In my opinion, it makes sense to change the diet frequently, with various cancer fighting foods, so the cancer never knows what is coming. Of course, that is just *my* theory and I'm sticking to it.

What are not included in this list are meat choices, because this list is intended to be the additives to go along with the meat of your choice. For human cancer warriors, meat is a big 'no-no,' because it is acidic and feeds cancer. For dogs, it's a little different, because their bodies need meat protein and I have read meat should make up approximately 40 percent of the protein, per meal, for canine cancer diets. I would alternate types of meat and use only high quality, grass fed, antibiotic and hormone free. Salmon is an excellent choice, because of the additional omega 3 fatty acids it will add to the diet, but make sure it is NOT farm raised. Wild Alaskan salmon didn't always fit our budget, so we mostly fed Nola antibiotic free, organic chicken. She was a big dog with a big appetite. Thankfully, she maintained a healthy appetite throughout her entire journey.

You should feed all fruits and vegetables raw or lightly steamed, when applicable, to get the most nutrients from them. They should be pureed, as I mentioned before, because it's hard for dogs to break down fruits and vegetables. Its digestive tract is much shorter than ours, which means most of the vegetable will end up in its poop before it can absorb the nutrients, if you don't break it down for them. Juicing is a great option too, but I would include some of the pulp into its food so it reaps the benefits of the fiber lost in the juicing process.

As for feeding your cancer dog raw meat, my opinion is it's great if you are already feeding raw. If you have never given it a raw diet and thinking of trying it, please do your research first. I wish I had more information on raw feeding to share, because there is strong evidence to support it is the healthiest way to feed dogs. I have not transitioned my dogs into a completely raw diet and, therefore, I can't give advice in this area. I do plan to research this more in the future and incorporate raw feeding into my current and future dogs' diets. I can only tell you I don't think it's as simple as handing them a raw chicken and letting them go to town. It's important to research this extensively before trying it, but I think it is worth the research. If you are not feeding raw now, I would not recommend you transition your cancer dog to raw meat, when you have so many other necessary changes to its diet. That is just my opinion; your holistic vet will have more advice for you in this area as well as the Yahoo groups. Following is my list of cancer fighting, immune building and alkalizing foods I fed Nola and I'm recommending for your cancer warrior:

Dark leafy greens are important for maintaining alkalinity in the body, as well as a great source of fiber, vitamins, minerals and protein. You should include some kind of dark leafy green into every meal. Following are our favorites, but you don't have to limit your choices to the ones on our list because there are so many from which to choose.

Kale – Kale is a great source of vitamins C, A, B-6, K, and folate as well as minerals such as iron and calcium. It's also a great source of fiber. Kale is the best bang for your buck for the small amount needed to reap the great benefits.

Spinach – Spinach has a high nutritional value and is extremely rich in antioxidants, especially when fresh, steamed, or quickly boiled. It is a rich source of vitamin A and especially high in lutein, vitamins C, B2, B6, E, K, magnesium, manganese, folate, betaine, iron, calcium, potassium, folic acid, copper, protein, phosphorus, zinc, niacin, selenium and omega-3 fatty acids. That last one should have caught your attention! Remember to oxygenate with as much Omega-3 as possible. (Source)

Romain lettuce – Romain lettuce is a very good source of dietary fiber and minerals such as manganese, potassium, copper, and iron and vitamins such as biotin, B1, and C.

Plant Proteins are a great way to enhance its food and satisfy your dog longer between meals, because of all the added nutrients and fiber. For human cancer patients, beans are typically the replacement for meat in a great cancer fighting diet. Dark leafy greens, mentioned before, are a good source of plant protein, but the following are even better:

Black Beans – Black beans are full of antioxidant and anti-inflammatory phytonutrients, which are very important in a good cancer fighting diet.

Garbanzo Beans – Like black beans, garbanzo beans are full of phytonutrients that have been proven to help fight cancer.

Green Beans – Green beans are loaded with nutrients and are a great source of vitamins K, C, A, manganese, fiber, potassium, folate and iron, thiamin, riboflavin, copper, calcium, phosphorus, protein, omega-3 fatty acids and niacin. Did I say omega-3? Yes, I did.

All beans are very good for dogs and a great source of plant protein.

Quinoa – Quinoa is one of the **best sources of plant protein,** iron and antioxidants. It is typically mistaken for a grain, but it is actually from the seed family. The seeds should always be soaked for a few hours and rinsed thoroughly, prior to cooking.

Other cancer fighting foods, that have been studied and proven to aid in healthy cell growth and to have cancer fighting properties, are listed below – **please note: if you are using Artemisinin, all of these foods, including the plant proteins, should be fed at least <u>five hours before</u> dosing the Artemisinin due to the high levels of iron and anti-oxidants in the food:**

Apples – One of the most delicious prescriptions ever made are apples. They are a powerful source of antioxidants, including polyphenols, flavonoids, and vitamin C, as well as a great source of fiber and potassium. They are great for juicing or just fed as an afternoon snack.

Beets – This quote was taken from an article on the study of beetroot by <u>The Underground Health Reporter,</u> "Science has proven beyond all doubt that a high intake of vegetables for cancer and fruits can reduce the risk of developing cancer and other disease. Beetroot in particular is extraordinarily rich in unique disease-fighting and anti-cancer chemicals.

The beautiful, rich crimson color of the beet comes from *betacyanins*, natural compounds that are powerful cancer-fighting agents. Beets also contain powerful health-promoting phytochemicals called *betalains*.

One of the most researched *betalains* in beets is called *betanin*. Betanin has outstanding anti-inflammatory, antioxidant, and detoxifying effects. According to The World's Healthiest Foods (a website run by the not-for-profit George Mateljan Foundation, devoted to fostering a healthier world), lab studies show that betanin pigments can impede tumor cell growth in tissues from the: Colon, Stomach, Nerves, Lungs, Breasts, Prostate & Testicles." Read more: http://undergroundhealthreporter.com/vegetables-for-cancer-beetroot/#ixzz3HemjaLy9

Berries – Blueberries, strawberries and raspberries are very high in antioxidants and have wonderful cancer fighting and alkalizing properties.

Braggs Raw Organic Apple Cider Vinegar – ACV promotes alkalinity. Remember, cancer cannot survive in an alkaline body. ACV is high in anti-oxidants and provides immune system support. It is great mixed with one teaspoon raw organic honey and bee pollen in a warm glass of water. You can use a food syringe to help your dog drink the water if it isn't willing on its own. If your dog is experiencing swollen lymph nodes, due to the cancer or other infections, ACV also works very well to clean out swollen lymph nodes. We experienced this with Nola one night when the lymph nodes all over her body started to swell, due to an infection she had acquired from her amputation surgery. The ACV worked within minutes and the swelling went down rapidly.

Broccoli – **Phytochemicals in broccoli can** boost DNA repair in cells **and may stop them from becoming cancerous.** It contains more vitamin C than an orange and it's a great source of potassium. Broccoli is also considered a great source of nutrients because it is rich in vitamin C, carotenoids (vitamin A-like substances), fiber, calcium, and folate. Broccoli releases the most nutrients when steamed for five minutes. Don't forget to puree it after you steam it.

Brussels sprouts – The following quote by Dr. Mercola in an article on Mercola.com supports the theory that Brussels sprouts are not only a great source of Vitamins C & K as well as B vitamins, fiber, potassium and manganese, but they also have wonderful cancer fighting properties. "Brussels sprouts contain sulfur-containing compounds called glucosinolates, which your body uses to make isothiocyanates, which activate cancer-fighting enzyme systems in your body. As reported in the journal *Carcinogenesis*:1"

Read more:

http://articles.mercola.com/sites/articles/archive/2014/05/12/brussels-sprouts.aspx.

All cruciferous vegetables are great for alkalinity and have cancer fighting properties.

Budwig diet – The Budwig diet was discovered by Dr. Budwig and has been used to treat cancer as well as other degenerated diseases with great success. It is one of the best ways to oxygenate the blood and it is so simple that it seems ridiculous it could have any benefit at all. Make no mistake, it is for real. Please do your own research before discounting the importance of this simple supplement into your daily regimen. The Budwig diet is simply flax seed oil blended with cottage cheese. That's it. You take three tablespoons flaxseed oil and six tablespoons low fat (less than 2%) cottage cheese and blend with a hand held immersion blender, until the oil has completely blended with the cottage cheese. It should take about two minutes. It's done when you no longer see any trace of oil, the mixture is creamy and the color turns slightly yellow or beige. After the blending is complete, only then can you add other foods, like berries or the greens mixture I describe in the chapter, *Cancer Fighting Menu*. Once the flax seed oil and cottage cheese are blended completely, the cottage cheese is no longer a dairy (science that I can't explain, but I trust that it is true). The combination of the two reacts in the body by flooding the bloodstream with oxygen. Those are my words, but that is the basic concept. If you want to learn all of the science behind it, you can Google, The Budwig Diet, and find many websites to explain the science. This mixture must be eaten immediately after blending, so there is no benefit to making extra, to store for later. Since cottage cheese & flax oil is recommended to give with the Artemisinin, Budwigs is a great way to oxygenate the blood at night when cancer is most active. **Just be sure to give the plain Budwig mixture, without any fruit or greens added, if giving it along with the Artemisinin**.

Carrots – Carrots are an excellent source of beta-carotene and contain high amounts of fiber. The Gerson Institute uses carrot juice in very high quantities as part of its main nutrition protocol for fighting cancer.

Celery – Celery is a great source of vitamin C, fiber, potassium, folic acid, vitamins B6, B1, B2, calcium and a rich source of dietary sodium. Celery also has anti-inflammatory properties, which we know is vital when fighting cancer.

Coconut Water, Milk and Oil – Coconut water is a great source of hydration and electrolytes, while aiding the body in alkalinity. I liked to give Nola small drinks of it throughout the day with a food syringe and she loved it. The medium chain triglycerides (MCT) in coconut oil and coconut milk are metabolized differently by taking a path through the liver on the way to the digestive tract and releasing a quick boost of energy. MCTs are extremely beneficial to cancer patients. This quote was taken from an article by The Coconut Research Center, "MCT are easily digested, absorbed, and put to use nourishing the body. Unlike other fats, they put little strain on the digestive system and provide a quick source of energy necessary to promote healing. There have been many other studies done on the use of MCT to shrink cancer tumors. This is important for patients who are using every ounce of strength they have to overcome serious illness or injury." Read more: http://www.coconutresearchcenter.org/article10612.htm

By combining generous amounts of coconut oil with ample amounts of omega-3 (see Vitamins & Supplements) we are basically supporting and following the guidelines of a Ketogenic Diet, without the fasting, which has been used to starve cancer cells for years. If you want to learn more about the Ketogenic Diet, you can start with this article called *Ketogenic Diet to Fight Cancer*, on the *Cancer Active* website http://www.canceractive. com/cancer-active-page-link.aspx?n=3117.

I did not consistently give Nola coconut oil until the last month of her life and this is another choice that I regret, as I should have started her on it immediately. I highly recommend you immediately start your dog on three tablespoons of coconut oil (any size dog) throughout the day, every day, and even more if it likes it and wants it, within reason. Coconut oil is one of those super foods that are simply healthy. It can, however, give it a full feeling, since it saturates the liver on the way to the digestive tract, which might make it hard to feed it the necessary cancer fighting meals. I waited until after Nola ate or mixed it directly into her food.

Cucumbers – Cucumber is an excellent source of silica, which is known to help promote joint health by strengthening the connective tissues. They are also rich in vitamins A, B1, B6, C & D, Folate, Calcium, Magnesium and Potassium. Cucumber promotes alkalinity while calming inflammation in the body. Great for juicing and adding into the powerhouse breakfast mix.

Ground Egg Shells – Ground Egg Shells can be used in place of a calcium supplement. Clean them well; dry them in the oven for five to ten minutes on 350 degrees, before grinding them into a fine powder. Sprinkle approximately 1 tablespoon into the food at a time.

Lemon – Lemon is a great source of vitamin C. It is beneficial to drink warm lemon water before bed on an empty stomach to cleanse the bloodstream and starve the cancer. You can use a food syringe to help your dog drink the water if it isn't willing on its own. The following morning, include a lot of vitamin packed vegetables (juicing is best) with antioxidants and omega-3 with the breakfast meal, so the cancer is forced to take in the vitamins (that cancer hates) before feeding on anything else. Lemon is great to include into the morning juice as well to boost the system. **When taking Artemisinin, you won't be able to give the lemon water at night because vitamin C will counter with it, but the Artemisinin will be working in a very similar way and you will still benefit to flood the bloodstream with vitamins early in the morning to further starve any cancer the Artemisinin missed the night before.**

Lime – Like lemons, limes are a great source of vitamin C. They also have antibiotic and anti-carcinogenic properties. This quote was taken from an article called *What Are the Benefits of Lime Juice?* on the Livestrong.com website, "Lime juice has potent anti-carcinogenic properties. J. Robert Hatherill Ph.D., a research scientist, writes that limes and other citrus fruit contain a variety of cancer-fighting compounds called flavonoids. Flavonoids are a family of naturally-occurring compounds found in many fruit and vegetables. In his book "Eat To Beat Cancer," he reports that the biological activity of citrus juice flavonoids have anti-cancer effects that prevent the invasion of cancer cells. These compounds also powerfully inhibit the growth of tumor cells. He notes that the juice has most cancer-fighting clout when it is drunk fresh."

Read more: http://www.livestrong.com/article/260168-what-are-the-benefits-of-lime-juice/

Milk Kefir – Probiotics are very important to include into your daily diet regimen because they provide your body with "good" bacteria that maintains a healthy gut, aides in digestion and boosts the immune system. This is just as important for your pets, especially since many of them only eat dry kibble food and don't get the type of bacteria their bodies might get while hunting in the wild. Milk Kefir is a natural probiotic and a great source of calcium, iron and antioxidants. In case you are nervous about feeding your dog a dairy product that can be hard on its digestive system, don't be. The fermentation process pre-digests the lactose, making it very easy on their digestive system and milk kefir contains more strains of bacteria and yeast than yogurt or water kefir, therefore less of it is needed to reap great benefits.

Mushrooms – Mushrooms of all kinds have cancer fighting and immune building properties. Depending on the availability in your area, you can alternate varieties. Crimini, white button, portabella and shitake mushrooms were the ones we used the most. Dr. Baker told us white button mushrooms also have anti-inflammatory benefits as well. Many people in the dog cancer groups also give their dogs AHCC (medicinal mushroom extract) in supplement form, which is shown to have cancer fighting properties. We never used AHCC in Nola's protocol, but that doesn't make it wrong to include into yours. We had to draw the line somewhere on supplements and this was one that didn't make it into our protocol. The Beta-1, 3D Glucan that I mention in the chapter, *Vitamins & Supplements*, was our choice for this type of immune building, cancer fighting supplement and I explain why later.

Olive Oil – Olive oil is a very healthy fat that appears to have cancer fighting properties. According to *Olive Oil Source*, "Studies show that olive oil may play a part in reducing rates or risk of some types of cancer, particularly colon, breast, ovarian, and prostate cancers."

Read more: http://www.oliveoilsource.com/page/cancer

Adding one tablespoon of olive oil to its food is a great way to add healthy fats as well as aiding alkalinity.

Oranges – We all know oranges are a good source of vitamin C, but they are also high in fiber and aid in alkalinity. They are perfect to include in the morning juice and should be given early in the day, if using Artemisinin, because vitamin C will counter with it.

Raw Organic Honey & Bee Pollen – One tablespoon of each daily will boost its immune system. I like to combine them with one tablespoon coconut oil and blend them together for a tasty treat. Raw organic honey can also be added to Braggs ACV. Nola loved it either way. Many are nervous about the sugar in honey, which is why I limit to one tablespoon daily. The benefits of raw honey for the immune system far outweigh the small amount of natural sugar. Remember, Mother Nature knows what she is doing and she was not messing around when she created our bees that make this magical nectar.

Sweet Potato – I read that sweet potatoes and pumpkin are so good for dogs that you should feed it to them every day, so I have been ever since – even to my healthy, cancer free dogs. Contrary to their name, sweet potatoes are actually low glycemic and work to stabilize blood sugars, making them perfect for diabetics too. They have potent antioxidants, which aid in healing & cancer prevention. They are a source of Vitamins A, C and B6 as well as a great source of fiber to help with loose stools. Canned Pumpkin is another great remedy for loose stools. **Please note: white potatoes are not the same as sweet potatoes and should not be given to cancer patients because they have a high glycemic rating, which means they quickly turn to sugar in the body. Remember, sugar feeds cancer.**

Zucchini – Zucchini is a good source of vitamins C, B6, riboflavin, and manganese, as well as a lot of other nutrients. It is great for juicing and adding into the powerhouse breakfast mix.

Dangerous Foods for Dogs

Following is a list of foods that may be healthy for humans, but are dangerous for dogs and should never be included into your cancer fighting diet or your healthy dog's diet, for that matter. I'm not going to list all of the reasons why they are dangerous, as you can easily research that information. I would concentrate on researching the healthy, cancer fighting foods and just trust that you should stay away from the following foods in your protocol for your canine cancer warrior:

Chocolate

Onions – please note that, although onions are a great cancer fighting food for humans, they are dangerous for dogs and cats.

Avocado

Macadamia nuts

Sugarless gum – keep out of reach as it's VERY DANGEROUS for dogs.

Grapes and raisins

Dairy (in high quantities)

You should always cross reference all "people foods" and research whether they are safe for dogs (or other animals) before feeding them to your pets. This is true for all supplements, herbs and spices.

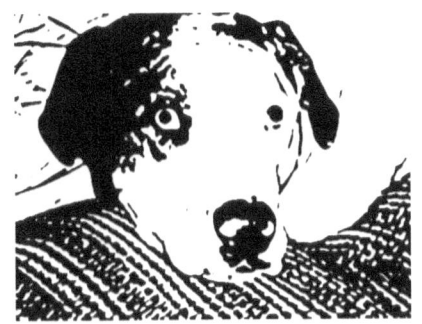

Medicinal Herbs & Spices

Herbs and spices have been used for their natural healing capabilities for centuries, but somewhere along the way they became "alternative" medicine. The truth is our pharmaceutical companies create medicines that try to mimic the properties of natural remedies our ancestors used from the earth hundreds of years ago. The difference being, the man made versions always come with side effects.

Following are the herbs and spices that made it into our final protocol. **If you are using Artemisinin, all of the following should be given at least five hours from the Arte due to the antioxidant properties in the herbs and spices that could counter the oxidants in the Artemisinin.**

Basil – Holy basil is considered to be the most sacred herb of India. It is now becoming more recognized, worldwide, for its disease fighting properties. According to *Natural Health 365*, "The active constituent in holy basil leaf, eugenol is responsible for its anticancer potential. It turns out that eugenol inhibits the multiplication, migration and invasion of cancer cells and will also induce apoptosis (programmed cell death of tumors). Furthermore, holy basil has a host of cancer-fighting phytochemicals like, apigenin, luteolin, rosmarinic acid, myretenal, beta-sitosterol and carnosic acid. According to a recent 2013 research published in Nutrition and Cancer, these compounds increased the antioxidant activity and destroyed cancer cells. It was shown that flavonoid compounds in water extracts of holy basil, orintin and vicenin protected mice against radiation-induced tumor." Read more: http://www.naturalhealth365.com/food_news/0897_holy_basil_cancer.html#sthash.O0j5UPbS.dpuf

Essiac Tea – Essiac Tea is something that came up often in the dog cancer Yahoo groups, but since I was already using Graviola Tea

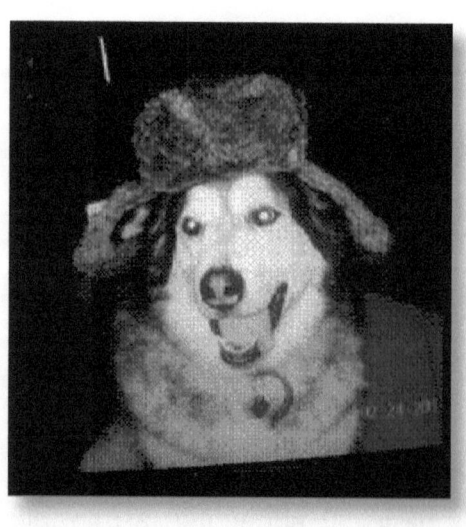

at the time, I decided that it wasn't important to change to Essiac. I could not have been more wrong. They are not even close and not incorporating Essiac into our protocol sooner is one of my biggest regrets. It wasn't until I had a conversation with my friend, Juli, from the Artemisinin group who had a 180lb Alaskan Malamute, Chalali (shown here), with OS in her hind leg that I realized the potential this tea has for slowing and curing cancer. Juli & Chalali were also fighting the cancer 100% naturally with wonderful success. Chalali was given the same estimate of three months to live upon the original diagnosis, which they turned into over two years! Further, due to Chalali's size, they never amputated! These are amazing results and proof that statistics are not worth worrying about because every dog and every situation is different.

I do want to add, although I met Juli in the Artemisinin Group, she only used Arte for a short period of time. Arte was one in a handful of natural treatments that she introduced all at once at the beginning of their fight. Chalali became very ill as a result (vomiting from heavy detoxification). They had to stop everything and introduce each treatment slowly and one at a time. Arte was never reintroduced, but she stayed in the group for the same reason that I remain a member – the support.

Juli and I compared notes a lot since we were using much of the same protocol, except that she was using more Traditional Chinese Medicine (TCM) remedies as well as Essiac Tea. I did not put much thought into it until one day when we began to discuss Essiac Tea in more detail and I realized that I had been grossly underestimating this little miracle discovered by Nurse

Rene Caisse (Caisse spelled backwards is Essiac). The book, _Essiac Essentials_, covers what exactly Essiac is, how it works and success stories that validate its worth. The authors, Sheila Snow & Mali Klein, worked closely with Rene Caisse when writing the book. I highly recommend you add it to your resource library if you plan to prepare the tea.

There are a lot of versions of Essiac tea on the market and some even provide it in a pill form for convenience. In my opinion, the pills are a waste of money because they do not follow the exact method of brewing the tea, that Rene Caisse used, and cutting corners for convenience will not bring you the same results. Make sure that the tea is created exactly like the concoction that Rene Caisse developed, which should include Burdock root, Sheep Sorrel (whole herbs plus roots), Slippery Elm inner bark & Turkey rhubarb **in the exact ratios stated in the book.** One company that was recommended to me by Juli and where I purchased my Essiac Tea is Essiac West. Later Juli discovered Rene Caisse Tea, http://renecaissetea.com/, whose owner works closely with Mali Klein. Another reputable company that Bill Henderson mentions in his book, _Cancer-Free: Your Guide to Gentle, Non-toxic Healing_, is Allen's Club, http://allensclub.com/, owned by Allen Wenzel. Mr. Wenzel has researched Essiac Tea for many years, including trips to Nurse Caisse's home town, and created a blend of the herbs which matches exactly Nurse Caisse's original formula.

I'm sure there are other reputable companies not mentioned here, but do your research and don't be afraid to pick up the phone and ask them for proof that their Essiac is made from Rene Caisse's formula or as close to it as possible. The other important factor to note is that it is very important to cook the tea exactly per the instructions in the book, *Essiac Essentials*. You must use stainless steel and/or glass pots, measuring cups and utensils and sterilize everything prior to making the tea. All of these steps are crucial as well as the time & temperature for which it is cooked. It is also important that you give the Essiac on an empty stomach and within an hour of any other food or water. The doses are small, only (1) Tbs, two to three times a day – starting with one, building up to two or three. A little goes a long way. Store the left over tea in sterilized dark glass containers and refrigerate.

This all sounds like a lot of work, which is partially why I didn't start Nola on the Essiac Tea sooner, but Juli swears by it and feels that the tea, diet, and homeopathy were the three most important treatments in her protocol. She felt that it gave Chalali an additional two years of life. After reading *Essiac Essentials*, I have to say that I believe there is strong evidence to back that up. If I had it to do over, Essiac Tea would be at the top of the list of my protocol from day one. I didn't start Nola on it until the last couple months of her journey after the cancer had already spread to her lungs.

<u>Garlic</u> – Garlic is a powerhouse of immune building, cancer fighting properties wrapped up in a tiny little bulb. It's a powerful anti-inflammatory and aids in pH alkalinity. Garlic is almost always found on the dangerous foods lists for dogs, but it has also been included into almost every canine cancer fighting diet that I have found on the internet, so I was very confused about the safety of garlic for dogs until I discussed it with Dr. Baker. She confirmed that garlic is completely safe and recommended it when given in moderation. The exact amount depends on the size of your dog and you should consult with your holistic vet for the proper dosing recommendation for your warrior.

With further research on the topic, I found that the reason why it shows up on the list is because garlic and onions contain thiosulphate, which is the substance that causes 'Heinx Factor' anemia in dogs and cats; therefore, they get grouped together as unsafe food for dogs and cats. But onions have a much higher amount of thiosulphate than garlic, which has almost untraceable amounts when given properly, and therefore cannot be compared to an onion with regard to toxicity for canines. **Cats, however, are much more sensitive to thiosulphate and should NOT have garlic or onions**. For dogs, garlic is a powerhouse of immune building, cancer fighting properties and should be included into your cancer fighting diet. I gave Nola one clove with every meal – up to three cloves per day. Again, she was an

80 pound dog with cancer. I currently give my healthy, medium-size dogs (30 – 45 lbs) – half a clove each, a few times a week, to boost their immune systems and keep their bodies alkaline. Being a great antibiotic as well, garlic helps minor scrapes heal faster, so I give them a daily dose for a few days if they get scraped up while playing outside.

Another reason why I am now a garlic endorser is because of the following story. Remember how Nola's rash cleared up almost overnight once I enhanced her diet? Well, when I was tracking her food charts, to see what I had done differently in the last few days that might have helped, I realized it was after I decided garlic was safe and added it to the diet. I was immediately convinced that not only was it safe, it was powerful.

To further ease your mind on feeding garlic to your dog; when giving Nola garlic, her blood work always came back perfect and her liver functions were always normal when checked. She never had any issues, nor do my healthy dogs that eat garlic on a regular basis. If, after reading this, you *still* have reservations about feeding garlic to your dog, then don't do it. I don't want to push someone into doing something that they fear is harmful to their pet and I want you to feel really good about all the decisions that you make for your cancer warrior.

<u>Ginger</u> – Georgia State University did a study to prove ginger destroys cancer more effectively than chemotherapy (<u>source</u>). Taken from another source, the following quote is from an article on the _Natural Society_ website called _Ginger Destroys Cancer More Effectively than Death-Linked Cancer Drugs_ by Anthony Guccairdi, "Ginger, a cousin spice of super anti-cancer substance turmeric, is known for its ability to shrink tumors. Astoundingly, it is even more effective than many cancer drugs, which have been shown to be completely ineffective and actually accelerate the death of cancer patients. Commonly consumed across the world in small doses among food and beverage products, the medicinal properties of ginger far surpass even advanced pharmaceutical inventions." – Read more: http://naturalsociety.com/ginger-destroys-cancer-more-effectively-than-cancer-drugs/#sthash.C3HR8UWR.dpuf

Ginger is also an amazing anti-inflammatory and promotes alkalinity in the body. A little ginger goes a long way and a small amount (1 tsp of fresh ginger, which is approximately 1/2" peeled and finely chopped) should be in every meal. You can also press it with a garlic press, which is my husband's preferred method.

<u>Parsley</u> – Most people think of parsley as the garnish on the side of the plate, but it has three times as much vitamin C as an orange and holds its own against spinach with the amount of iron it provides. The most important reasons to include a little parsley

into every meal – it's alkalizing, it's a great anti-inflammatory and it contains volatile oils that have been found to inhibit tumor formation.

Turmeric – <u>Phytochemicals found in turmeric</u> have been researched for their potential effects on cancer and other diseases. Turmeric has long been used as a powerful anti-inflammatory in both the Chinese and Indian systems of medicine. **Always use turmeric in conjunction with fresh ground black pepper because the pepper increases the efficacy (absorption into the body) of the turmeric.** The natural fat in coconut oil will also increase absorption, so the trio is unrivaled in your fight against cancer. I highly recommend adding a teaspoon into every meal with several dashes of black pepper and a spoon full of coconut oil – I can't say enough about the importance of this spice for a complete cancer fighting diet.

<u>Wheatgrass</u> – Wheatgrass juice contains approximately 70% chlorophyll which means it is a blood builder. It is also high in oxygen and therefore another great way to oxygenate the blood and starve cancer cells. You will get the most benefits from fresh wheatgrass juice, which requires a special wheatgrass juicer. If you are not able to purchase a wheatgrass juicer, your second best method is to add wheatgrass powder to your dog's food. It may not get the full 70% chlorophyll as it would with fresh wheatgrass juice, but some is better than none.

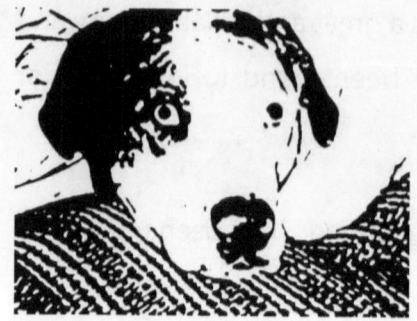

Vitamins & Supplements

Although it's important to obtain most of the vitamins and nutrients through clean food, a well rounded cancer fighting protocol *does* include specific vitamins and supplements to fill in the gaps. It's especially necessary when fighting cancer 100% holistically because some of these supplements will take the place of chemotherapy or enhance it if you choose to do both.

Following is my recommendation of the most important vitamins and supplements that made it into our final protocol - some of them a little too late. **I <u>don't</u> recommend you start all of these at one time**. It's best to introduce each supplement, one at a time, for a couple reasons. If it has a bad reaction to something, you immediately know what is causing the reaction – the same is true for a good response. If your dog shows great improvement, you want to know exactly which supplement, or combination of supplements, is working. Most importantly, it's easier on its system to introduce them one at a time. I would leave several days, even a week, before adding each one. Some of these, such as the vitamins, are okay to combine together at once from the beginning. You should use common sense as well as the advice of your veterinarian for dosage recommendations on all vitamins and supplements.

Artemisinin –Artemisinin is a gentle, non-toxic, natural supplement that has proven to work well against many types of cancer cells. It is an oxidant that attaches to the iron in cancer cells and kills them. It's important to feed a low dose of vitamin C & E the morning after you dose the Arte to clean the bloodstream of the dead cancer cells that were killed by the Arte the night before. All other antioxidants and iron should also be given early in the morning, as far away from the Arte consumption as possible, because antioxidants will cancel it out (since it is an oxidant) and you want the Arte to attach to the iron in the cancer cells and not to the iron from the food.

Don't feed your warrior anything *at least* five hours prior to dosing the Artemisinin, to ensure that there isn't any iron (from food) lingering in the bloodstream. This might mean setting your alarm to get up if your dog is a late eater, like Nola was. I had to set my alarm for 1:00 am many times.

Artemisinin should be given along with Butyrex and a small amount of natural fat, such as cream cheese, cottage cheese or yogurt, because it has been proven to help with the efficacy of the Arte. Fish oil and flax seed oil are also beneficial to give along with Arte, **which makes Budwigs a great cohort to the cancer killing combo**, **at night when cancer is most active** - the bloodstream gets a hit of oxygen from the Budwig's to starve the cancer cells, while the Arte attaches to the cancer and kills it. Knowing this always made me sleep a little better.

Another easy option for feeding the Arte is to hide the pills in little balls of cream cheese, which every dog seems to love. It isn't as healthy of an option, but the natural fat works well with the Arte and it is much easier (and tastier) to feed to your dog, especially at 1:00 am for those late eaters. I would make up the balls ahead of time and keep them by the bed, so I just had to reach over and feed them to her when my alarm went off. She thought it was awesome that I set an alarm, just to get up and give her a tasty treat. Win/win for both of us.

Sometimes I gave Nola Budwigs <u>without greens</u> as her latest meal with very little meat so that she still got the burst of oxygen late at night and I didn't have to wait the full 5 hours to give her the Arte with cream cheese (still waited at least 4 if I fed chicken). This seemed to work well and was the best of both worlds with plenty of natural fat and the easy late night administering of the Arte.

You can use the cream cheese trick with all of the pills that go with the Arte, (Butyrex & fish oil). Once you join the <u>Artemisinin Yahoo</u>

Group, you will learn so much more information on Artemisinin and its derivatives and dosage recommendations for your dog. This is a very safe, holistic cancer killer that I highly recommend you begin as soon as possible. If your vet is not familiar with this supplement, bring him or her up to speed as quickly as you can. Another great secondary benefit of Arte is that it is made from wormwood, which is a natural parasite killer and will help to prevent heartworms and other parasites since you should not treat your cancer dog with harsh chemicals.

Astragalus – Astragalus is commonly used with Traditional Chinese Medicine (TCM) for various reasons, but immune system support is at the core of it. I recommend two 500mg pills per day – this should be ¼ of the amount of the human dosage unless you have a very large breed dog, which can handle a full human dosage.

The following information about Astragalus was quoted from the Memorial Sloan Kettering Cancer Institute's website, "Astragalus has been studied for its anticancer potential but evidence is limited. Astragalus extracts were shown to inhibit tumor growth... Use of an injectable form of Astragalus with vinorelbine and cisplatin in patients with advanced non-small cell lung cancer (NSCLC) [20] resulted in improvement in quality of life. However, it is not known whether orally administered Astragalus will exert the same effects. In another study, an Astragalus extract was found effective in managing cancer-related fatigue." More information can be found at http://www.mskcc.org/cancer-care/herb/astragalus.

Avemar (Shield4Pets) – You can find a lot of information that explains how Avemar works on the Shield4Pets website, (http://www.shield4pets.com/), but I will narrow down the main points in layman's terms. Basically Avemar (Shield4Pets) does two things in the body that are significant for fighting cancer. First, it increases the number of fighter cells in the body that actually go out and find cancer cells to kill, therefore building the army and enhancing the immune system. Second, it makes it impossible for the cancer cells to camouflage themselves as healthy cells, which cancer cells will eventually achieve.

Cancer cells are smart and they somehow figure out ways to trick the body into thinking they are healthy cells. Avemar helps the body to always recognize them as cancer cells. There is scientific evidence that explains how and why this happens that you will find in the information provided on the Shield4Pets website.

The following quote was taken from an article on Avemar (included in the appendix), "Avemar is fermented wheat germ that has been put through many different processes to achieve its remarkable capabilities. It was discovered in Hungary where it is widely used but now is also gaining acceptance in the United States. Memorial

Sloan Kettering Cancer Institute has been recognizing the value of this product in treating cancer patients. I'll try to explain how it works but it works in many different ways, on a cellular level to destroy cancer cells or at the least, to remove their ability to thrive."

The only way to purchase Shield4Pets is from Barbara Bouyet, an angel in our midst that has given up a lot to import Avemar into the US under the name Shield4Pets, so that our pets will have the opportunity and access to this amazing supplement.

There have been many trials and tribulations for Barbara, to make this product available to us, and she makes very little profit for all of her efforts. She is not in it for the money and she makes this clear by all of her hard work on our behalf for so little. Her payment comes from all of the feedback she gets from the pet owners that swear by the results after giving Shield4Pets to their sick animals. Shield4Pets is the exact same product that they use in Hungary, under the name of Avemar, which has become part of their regular practice for their human cancer patients. This product is especially important to give your pet if it is undergoing chemotherapy and radiation, as it has been shown to help with the success in the treatments.

There are no harmful side effects while giving this product along with chemo or radiation as well as any other medications. The only conflict noted is with vitamin C in the form of ascorbic acid. You should not give Vitamin C within two hours of Avemar (Shield4Pets) because it can cause it to be less effective.

Nola's cancer did not metastasize to her lungs until I eventually took her off of this product due to financial reasons. It was about a month after I made that choice that her cancer spread from her leg to her lungs. I'm not saying that it wouldn't have happened had I left her on the Shield4Pets, because I will never know. It is something that I ask myself a lot. If I had it to do over, I would have definitely left her on the Shield4Pets and done without something else. The great news is the price for Shield4Pets has been greatly reduced since Nola was sick and now it is affordable to purchase for your healthy pets too, for cancer prevention and immune support.

Bromelain – Bromelain is not only a great anti-inflammatory, but research is also showing that the protease enzymes that Bromelain contains also have an anti-cancer nutrient support. According to Byron J. Richards, Board certified clinical nutritionist, in the _Wellness Resources_ article called, _Bromelain Has Potent Anti-Cancer Properties_, "A recent study on human cancer cells showed that Bromelain could act directly to kill cancer cells[3] and was possibly more than just a support for other cancer therapies. It directly knocked out the core aberrant gene signal, NF-kappaB, along with the inflammation that is typical in cancer. On the other hand, within the cancer cells themselves, it unleashed massive free radical damage that caused the cancer cells to die (something it does not do to healthy cells)." Read more, http://www.wellnessresources.com/health/articles/bromelains_potent_anti-cancer_properties_identified/

I only stumbled upon Bromelain toward the end, once Nola's tumor began to fracture the bone in her leg. Bromelain came up in my research as a great supplement for broken bones – both with inflammation and for bone formation. Since I always did a cross reference to see if my natural pain supplements were also good for fighting cancer, I discovered that Bromelain was great for fighting cancer cells. Bromelain is another supplement that I would have started Nola on right away if I had known about it sooner because it is also very inexpensive.

Pineapple is a great source of Bromelain, but I recommend the Bromelain supplements because your dog would need to eat a lot of pineapple to get the recommended dosage of Bromelain. That doesn't mean you can't also include a little pineapple into your dog's diet as well.

The next three supplements, (1)BETA-1,3D Glucan, (2)Heart Plus with Green Tea Extract, and (3)Dried Green Barley, were added toward the end of my research when I discovered a book called *Cancer-Free: Your Guide to Gentle, Non-toxic Healing* by Bill Henderson, which I hope you will add to your resource library too.

Mr. Henderson has provided one of the best resources for anyone fighting cancer naturally, as well as their caregivers. I used his book like my bible, during our fight. I cross referenced the supplements he suggests in his book, to ensure the supplements I incorporated into our protocol were safe for canines. This is the main reason why I decided to create this resource for other canine cancer warriors. I've already done the work, why not share it? As I mentioned before, I stumbled upon this book toward the end of my research and it filled in the final missing pieces to our protocol. I only wish I had found it sooner in our journey.

I had already incorporated into our protocol many of the things Mr. Henderson mentions in his book, which was a wonderful confirmation that my research had lead me to many great decisions. However, these last three supplements were missing and I believe they are all among the most important additions that came too late in our battle.

BETA-1, 3D Glucan – In my opinion, this is the very best option for an immune building supplement. The company from which to purchase the BETA-1,3D Glucan is www.betterwayhealth.com/. You can find less expensive options of BETA-1 Glucan at the health food store, but it will not be the same product. I wrote to Reggie Black at BetterWay Health to thank him for always including a hand written *thank you* note with every order and to ask him questions about the product. He replied back to me with a lot of helpful information. You will find that many people in the dog cancer groups will be using and recommending K9 Immunity with Transfer Factor, which we also used until I found this product.

The BETA-1,3D Glucan may seem like a more expensive option, but you only have to dose it once in the morning, no matter the size of your dog, and the K9 Immunity is administered by weight, which means you have to give a lot more pills to larger dogs, while you are already giving them so many different pills throughout the day. When I asked Mr. Black the question about how the BETA-1,3D Glucan compared to the K9 Immunity with Transfer Factor, following was his email back to me.

> Heather:
>
> I apologize for the late response. I had your email marked as important and was intending to gather some research for you and send it back. Better late than never right?
>
> I attached 3 documents for you for specific research comparing our product to Transfer Factor. Keep in mind as well that this was an animal study (lab rats) so the immune system of your dog and the mice is going to be very similar.

-The first is a visual - Beta Glucan Tower - The results of the study done at University of Louisville and published in the journal of the American Nutraceutical association in 2008. Our product was found to the best supplement tested among hundreds of the most popular immune system supplements. As you can See the 4life immune supplement is on the bottom.

-The 2nd JANA2008 is the actual published study where you can view the testing methods and processes done to reach these results.

-The 3rd is basically the same results but in a text form. As you can see here Transfer Factor was shown to have the same effect as the salt water during the test. It is hard to argue with science that proves their product is junk. But they do a great job marketing.

Please let me know if you have any more ?'s I would love to help out in any way I can

Thank You,
Reggie Black
BetterWayHealth.Com

2440 Sandy Plains Road Bld 24 Suite
300, Marietta, Georgia 30066
Phone: 800.746.7640 - Fax 678.567.9271 -
https://www.betterwayhealth.com

I should clarify that I believe Mr. Black didn't realize we were giving the Transfer Factor along with the K9 Immunity, only as support because Transfer Factors are proteins your dog naturally produces and they join with other immune-specific molecules to create antibodies. It was recommended to give this along with the K9 Immunity to boost the efficacy in the body, but unfortunately this means even more pills on a daily basis to achieve results that aren't as good as the BETA-1,3D Glucan, which is a far superior product in my opinion. I have included all three documents that he mentions in his email, in the appendix.

Vitamin C/Lysine/Proline (Heart Plus) & Green Tea Extract — Following is a quote by Bill Henderson from his book, *Cancer-Free: Your Guide to Gentle, Non-toxic Healing,* "This combination [Vit C/Lysine/Proline] was discovered by Dr. Matthias Rath and Dr. Linus Pauling in the mid-1980's. They later strengthened this compound by adding green tea extract, finding that it improved the effect by about 30%. They found that this combination **inhibited the process of metastasis of cancer cells**. You can study this concept in detail at Dr. Rath's website: http://www4.dr-rath-foundation.org/pdf-files/cancerresearch.pdf

If you have cancer, one of your first priorities is to **slow down or stop the process of metastasis** (spreading of cancer cells to other parts of the body). Metastasis and its effect on organs, blood, brain, bone marrow, etc. is what kills cancer patients."

You can read more about the study in Mr. Henderson's book or the link I mentioned above. Since Dr. Rath's version of this compound is very expensive (even though all of the ingredients are inexpensive, abundant and readily available), Mr. Henderson worked with Our Health Coop, which is a company that sells their supplements for wholesale+5%, to create a more affordable version. The Vitamin C/Lysine/Proline is sold as Heart Plus (because it is also effective in preventing heart disease) and the Green Tea Extract is sold separately, since Dr. Rath has a patent on the combination - all in one pill.

Mr. Henderson recommends (for fighting cancer) taking (6) Heart Plus (2-2-2) throughout the day along with (3) (1-1-1) Green Tea Extract. You will find that the quantity of pills in the Heart Plus bottles and Green Tea Extract bottles work out perfectly if dosed as two Heart Plus for every one Green Tea Extract. After discovering Mr. Henderson's book, I gave Nola this recommended dosage for the duration of her journey. I also buy these for my mom, who has a history of heart issues, and she takes one dose of each per day.

My husband and I also take one dose per day for prevention. An interesting thing happened about a month after I started giving them to both my mom and my husband. They both asked me (at completely different times, not knowing the other one had asked me the same question) "Can you tell me again what is in these pills you are giving me and what they do?" When I asked why, they both responded with the exact same comment, "I'm not sure if it is the pills, but since I started taking them, I have noticed I feel really good. I think it's the pills because that is the only thing I have changed in my diet."

I have never determined exactly why the pills are making them both feel, "really good," or exactly what that means, but I thought it was worth sharing. If I had to guess, I think it's because the combination builds collagen in the body, which breaks down as you age. By replenishing it, it would most likely make you feel younger, which in turn could be described as, "feeling really good." I also want to mention this is also how it slows metastasis, because cancer breaks down collagen, which is how it spreads, so the Heart Plus/Green Tea re-builds the collagen, therefore inhibiting the process of metastasis.

Dried Green Barley – Mr. Henderson shared a story about Bob Davis and his experience with Barley Power by Green Supreme, explaining how it cured Bob's cancer along with his wife's arthritis.

If you didn't already know, cancer and arthritis are very similar in the way they survive and thrive in the body and neither is able to thrive in an alkaline environment. Enzyme Therapy is unrivaled at creating alkalinity in the body and is crucial to your cancer fighting protocol. Mr. Henderson quotes, "There are over 3,000 different types of enzymes in our bodies. Interestingly enough, the stuff that cured Bob Davis' cancer, green barley, contains all 3,000 of them, according to the discoverer, Dr. Yoshihide Hagiwara.," _Cancer-Free: Your Guide to Gentle, Non-toxic Healing_.

If you want to learn more about Enzyme Therapy or dried green barley pills and Bob Davis' success story, feel free to contact Bob at ACTS@interhop.net. I am sharing this information as it was given in Mr. Henderson's book, but I have not actually contacted Bob myself. I have, however, had many conversations with Green Supreme about Barley Power and they are extremely helpful and knowledgeable on the topic. They will also work with cancer patients on a payment plan and discounted bulk pricing, which they extended to Nola, even though she was a canine cancer patient. You can contact them at www.greensupreme.net/ or call 1-800-358-0777.

An important point both Bob and Mr. Henderson made about the dried green barley pills and enzyme therapies in general, is to take enough for them to work. You will start with (4) pills a day and gradually work up to at least (20) pills a day for them to be effective in killing cancer. This may sound like a lot until you see the pills. They are kind of like kibble dog food - they are a natural food supplement, not a pharmaceutical, so it really isn't a lot of pills when you think of it in terms of a food supplement.

You are supposed to take the pills with water approximately 20 minutes before eating, but if you can't get your dog to take them easily, you can always grind them up with a mortar and pestle and add them to the food.

Nola actually loved them and munched on them as a snack, but my two current (picky) dogs don't care for them, so I grind them and occasionally add them to their food, to prevent arthritis and cancer. They are still getting all of the beneficial enzymes that are important, especially as they age. Nola could have known this was something her body needed at the time, in the same way that dogs eat grass. My current healthy dogs may not feel they have a need for them yet. Always listen to your dogs, since they instinctively know what their bodies need.

I typically stay away from products people claim to be the next cancer cure or ultimate immune booster. This is an easy trap to fall into because you will run into a lot of these sales pitches, especially when researching canine cancer treatments. I prefer to rely on individual ingredients, provided by Mother Nature, to do what they are naturally designed to do. When in doubt, go back to the basics and make your own combinations, depending on the specific needs of your dog. That being said, I made exceptions to my rule with the three supplements above, because Mr. Henderson did extensive research to find them and has confirmed these products do exactly what they claim to do. I trust his opinion and sometimes you have to follow your gut.

If you want to learn more about these studies, Mr. Henderson goes into much greater detail explaining the science behind the products in his book, _Cancer-Free: Your Guide to Gentle, Non-toxic Healing_. I gave you my short hand version of the science, because my goal with this book is to break it down and attempt to simplify a massive amount of information. I also want to note neither Mr. Henderson, nor I receive any gifts or other payments from these companies or any other company I may mention. He makes this very clear in his book and I am doing the same in mine, because it is important to me you know I am only recommending them because I believe they play an important role in your protocol. My only agenda is to share what I have learned.

I can attest to the service and professionalism of all three of these companies after ordering from them and using their products. They are all very kind and helpful with questions, providing you with much needed information about their products as well as one-on-one attention when necessary. It is comforting knowing there is a real person behind the company whom you can call or email at any time.

Fish Oil – Fish oil is a great source of omega-3 and vital in oxygenating the blood to starve cancer cells. I started Nola (80 lb dog) on 4 pills a day and later learned in the Artemisinin Yahoo Group that the recommended dosage is 1000mg for every 10 lbs, so I doubled her dosage to 8-10 pills a day. Toward the end of our journey, I had a conversation with a gentleman who was doing extensive research on the Ketogenic Diet, utilizing MCT and Omega 3, and he informed me that I could and should be giving Nola up to 20,000mg a day for an 80 lb dog. That is what we gave her toward the end of her protocol and I really wished that I would have learned this sooner. I did get the approval from Dr. Baker, prior to doubling her dosage for the second time, and she explained that it takes very large doses of omega-3, when using it to oxygenate the blood for cancer treatment.

Some dogs will get soft or runny stool if given too much fish oil too quickly. If this happens, just back off to a smaller dose and try to slowly increase it over time, finding that sweet spot for your dog. We never had that issue with Nola and it might be because I increased it over time, but the increase wasn't what I would call gradual, since I doubled the dose with each increase. She was on each dosage for at least a couple months before it was doubled. If you have issues with diarrhea, you can add canned pumpkin or sweet potato to their food, which works like a charm to firm up soft stool.

Vitamin C – Dogs, unlike humans, create their own vitamin C and healthy dogs should not be given high doses of Vitamin C because their body may stop making it on its own. A cancer dog is different because they need the extra vitamin C to aid in healthy cell growth and building their immune system. There have been many studies on using large doses of vitamin C to treat cancer in humans. If you choose to use the Heart Plus supplements (Vitamin C/Lysine/Proline) with Green Tea then you will get more than enough vitamin C. You should not incorporate any other vitamin C supplements into your protocol, especially if given Heart Plus up to 3 times daily, which is the recommended dosage. If you are using Artemisinin, make sure that you leave a large window (5 to 6 hours minimum) before dosing the Artemisinin because of the antioxidant properties of Vitamin C and Green Tea, which will most likely mean that you can only give the Vitamin C/Lysine/ Proline with the Green Tea twice daily, which will be fine.

Vitamin D – Vitamin D is especially important for dogs with bone cancer, but not limited to bone cancer. Vitamin D increases the amount of calcium that is absorbed from food and is vital for bone formation, so when you are feeding them all of those wonderful dark leafy greens, you want the vitamin D to help the body absorb as much calcium from them as possible. It is also important for the regulation of cell growth, fighting infections, and immune function.

Vitamin E – The following quote was taken from the article, _Food for Life by Physicians Committee for Responsible Medicine_, "Its major function in the body is to act as an antioxidant. Vitamin E works quickly and reacts with destructive substances called free radicals, rendering them harmless before they get a chance to harm DNA, therefore preventing mutations and tumor growth." Read more: http://pcrm.org/health/cancer-resources/diet-cancer/nutrition/how-vitamin-e-helps-protect-against-cancer

It is important to give a low dose of Vitamin E in the morning when dosing Artemisinin at night to help the body discard all of the dead cancer cells that were killed throughout the night from the Artemisinin.

Multi-Vitamin – included into your daily routine should be a well rounded canine multi-vitamin. You can talk to your vet about his or her favorite brand or ask others in the Yahoo cancer groups. There are so many on the market and I don't have a favorite to recommend. As long as it's from a reputable company and has an all inclusive list of the necessary vitamins and minerals, it should be sufficient. If you follow my diet protocol, your dog will be getting most of its vitamins through its food, but a multi-vitamin supplement will fill in any gaps.

Vascu-Statin / C-Statin - is bindweed extract, also called Convolvulaceae, which has been proven to prevent cancer tumors from growing or spreading because of its anti-angiogenesis properties. This means that it inhibits angiogenesis, which is a process that restrains tumor blood vessel formation. Tumor formations must have a strong vascular system to survive, so by restraining the blood vessels, bindweed prevents tumors from forming. For this same reason, an animal or human with a heart condition should not take C-Statin (Vascu-Statin). I didn't learn about C-Statin until Nola had acquired lung mets. I learned that C-Statin can work well to keep the lung mets from spreading too quickly. After doing more research on bindweed, I believe it could have prevented the tumor from spreading to her lungs in the first place. This is why I am including Vascu-Statin into your daily protocol from the beginning.

Bindweed can be dosed at very high amounts without being toxic and we gave Nola (80 pounds) up to four pills three times a day. This was at a point where her cancer was very advanced, so we were hitting it hard. I think you could start with half that amount and build up over time, as necessary.

I recently learned the body's response to C-Statin is increased when given with Muramyl Polysaccharide-Glycan Complex (MPGC). We did not incorporate MPGC into our protocol because we did not have this information in time. I would combine the C-Statin with the MPGC, which is also non-toxic at high doses, to get the best response. You can purchase both products at Aidan Products

http://www.aidanproducts.com/products.html. The Bindweed is sold as C-Statin and the MPGC is sold as ImmKine at this company.

Giving pills to animals is not an easy task, so I developed a few tricks that worked well for us. I was lucky Nola was pretty good about taking pills, but with the amount of pills she had to take every day, I still changed it up throughout the day to keep her interested.

The easiest way is to hide the pill in its food. I opened a lot of her capsules and emptied them directly in the bowl, but you should do this with caution. I ruined an entire batch of food by adding Boswellia Extract and White Willow Bark to the food. It tasted disgusting. Since then, I always do a little sampling of the flavor of the powder in the capsule before adding it to the food. If it has a strong or bitter taste, I give the capsule whole. No supplements are going to taste great to us, but dogs actually like some of the "musty" or "earthy" tasting powders. It also depends on how picky your dog is and whether it does a smell test before eating.

Nola would eat almost anything I put in front of her, but the two dogs I have now, Barley and Suri, smell everything thoroughly and turn their noses up if they detect anything that doesn't smell "good" to them. They both like fish, so I always add a little canned tuna or salmon into their food when I need to make sure they eat every bite. The smell of the fish overrides anything else I might have hid into the mix.

The trick that I mentioned with the cream cheese balls, for dosing Artemisinin, works for any pill. I like this option because it makes your dog believe it is getting a tasty treat instead of a nasty pill. It helps to take a bad situation and turn it into a pleasurable one for them. One concern with this solution is the cream cheese, if given too much throughout the day, can be filling, causing your dog to not eat its healthy food. This is especially true if your dog is experiencing a loss of appetite from the illness or from pain. Another concern is the dairy can be hard for your dog to digest. For these reasons, I don't recommend this option to administer all its pills. I only used the cream cheese trick with the Artemisinin and the Tramadol (I discuss Tramadol in the chapter, *Pain Management*). The Artemisinin needs the natural fat and the Tramadol tastes horrible, making it hard to get your dog to swallow it without the cream cheese. Yes, I did a taste test on that too.

Sometimes you have to bite the bullet and shove the pills down their throat, gently of course. I got really good at this and had a system that seemed to be quick and painless for both of us. First, I noticed that Nola's mouth and throat were very dry and sticky if she had been sleeping or hadn't eaten recently. This made it almost impossible to get the pills to go down. I would always start by giving her a few drinks of water with a food syringe to moisten her throat. If your dog has just eaten or drank water, then this step is not necessary. I would then slide my thumb on my left hand (I'm right handed) into the side of her mouth, toward the back of her tongue, and gently held her tongue down with my thumb. While holding down her tongue, I placed the pill as far back into her throat as possible with my right hand, in a very quick motion. I then held her mouth closed, again gently, and blew in her nose lightly, which is supposed to cause them to swallow. You can also give your dog another drink with the syringe to wash the pill down. Lastly, I would ALWAYS follow up with a big smooch on the nose. That last step is the most important.

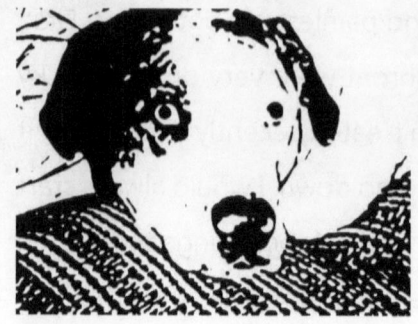

Cancer Fighting Menu

THREE SQUARES A DAY –
Breakfast, Snack & Dinner

The items I recommend to make this process easier are a blender, food processor and/or juicer, your favorite sharp chopping knife, a large cutting board, strainer with very small holes (for quinoa), large colander (for washing large amounts of fresh vegetables) and a hand held immersion blender (for Budwigs).

Following is the diet protocol we developed for Nola, but you will need to adjust feeding times and quantities per your dog's size, appetite and feeding routine. Nola was an 80 pound dog and she liked to eat three times a day, as a senior dog. As a younger dog, she only ate twice a day and my current dogs also only eat twice a day and sometimes only once a day. As Nola got older, we added a third, smaller meal (per her request) in the middle of the day that we considered a "snack" to satisfy her until dinner. This is why her cancer diet protocol includes the mid day snack, which your dog may not need or want.

It isn't important you follow this exact menu to the letter, as long as you include the same ingredients and make sure every bite of food that goes into its body has cancer fighting, alkalizing and anti-inflammatory properties. Your dog will let you know how much it can handle. Keep an eye out for a dramatic loss of appetite because this could be a sign of pain, among other things. Always consult your veterinarian if this occurs for more than a day.

Early Morning, prior to any other food and water – your first dose (1 tbs) of Essiac Tea should be given on an empty stomach and at least one hour before meals or supplements.

In my opinion, the most important component of Nola's meal for breakfast and dinner is what I call **Budwigs with Greens – see Budwig's Diet under *Nutrition ~ Mother Nature provides the best medicine,* for the directions for the Budwigs portion of this recipe**. **Note that the Budwigs mixture should be completely blended alone first before adding the vegetables, garlic and ginger.** This mixture will create an oxygen enriched gravy that is mixed into the rest of the dish. Don't forget to hold some back for yourself! It is delicious and it makes a great salad dressing.

Budwigs with Greens = one serving size of Budwig's mixture (see Budwig's Diet) mixed with a combination of puréed leafy greens, cruciferous vegetables, fresh herbs, one clove of garlic and ½" of peeled fresh ginger. It is great to have a different combination of vegetables all the time. It isn't an exact science - just use what you have on hand and make sure your kitchen is always stocked with a variety of clean, organic vegetables. For Nola's Budwigs with Greens, we used a variety of the following: romaine lettuce, kale, spinach, Brussel sprouts, cucumbers, celery, beets, broccoli, lemon, lime, parsley and basil. I prefer to have at least three different vegetable items from the list in each mixture. The mixture may become runny, depending on what type of vegetables you use. I try to include at least one cruciferous vegetable, to maintain thicker gravy (like coleslaw), so the overall food consistency isn't too runny. Sometimes that isn't possible, if the right vegetables aren't available, which does not mean it's not as healthy. If this happens, make your mid-afternoon snack a little heartier to make up for it, if your dog seems hungrier than normal. As I mentioned before, Nola had a big appetite, so the runnier meals did not satisfy her for long. A baked sweet potato makes a great, hearty mid-afternoon snack.

Note: On evenings that Artemisinin was given, I used a very small amount of vegetables in the Budwigs with Greens mixture and I fed Nola <u>no later</u> than 6:30pm. If it was necessary to feed her later than 6:30pm, I only added the Budwigs mixture <u>without the greens or garlic,</u> due to the high levels of iron and antioxidants that will affect the

efficacy of the Artemisinin. The same rule applies to the afternoon sweet potato mentioned above, due to its high antioxidant properties.

Following is a sample of a menu for one day's worth of meals and supplements for Nola, but the idea is that you will alternate meats and vegetables from the list in the nutrition section and hold the same rules for spacing high anti-oxidant and iron rich foods at least 5 hours (minimum) from the Artemisinin. Since Nola liked to eat pretty late, I had to set an alarm to get up to give her the Artemisinin at 12:30 am or sometimes 1:00 am. I did not include any pain medications or natural NSAIDS on the list because they will vary for your dog. This list includes all of the cancer fighting and immune building supplements that we gave her.

Breakfast – between 8:30am and 10:00am: - mix the following FOOD and SUPPLEMENTS together into a bowl. Again, this is based on an 80 pound dog with a hearty appetite.

FOOD:

(1 cup to 2 cups) cooked (boiled) organic chicken breasts
(1 serving) Budwigs with Greens – poured over chicken like a gravy
(½ cup) cooked quinoa (can be cooked ahead of time and stored in the refrigerator)

(3) fresh mushrooms chopped (any variety)

(1/3) baked sweet potato

(1/4 cup) beans – any variety

(1) fresh garlic clove - crush first, wait 5 min then chop finely or mince in garlic press

(1/2 inch) fresh ginger – peel and chop finely (or mince in press) (approx 1 tsp)

(1tsp) turmeric.

SUPPLEMENTS:

(4 tbs) Shield4Pets powder

(1) Astragalus pill (500 mg) – open capsule and pour into food if desired

(1 tbs) wheat grass powder

(2 tbs) coconut oil

(5) fish oil pills (1000 mg each)

(1) Vitamin E pill (200 mg each)

(2) D3 vitamin pill (1000 IU each)

(1 tbs) ground egg shells (or 1 calcium supplement)

(1 to 2 tbs) bee pollen (I just shake some in – no exact measurement needed)

(5) Dried Green Barley Pills (increase over time depending on your dog's weight and tolerance – Nola gets 5 or 6 at a time for a total of 15 to 20 a day). **Give the Dried Green Barley pills 20**

minutes before the rest of the meal, which follows the dosing guideline provided by Green Supreme.

(2) Beta 1, 3D Glucan pills. **Give the Beta 1, 3D Glucan pills 30 minutes before the rest of the meal since they are to be given 30 minutes before a meal. Beta 1, 3D Glucan are to be given only once daily in the morning.**

Note: (2) Heart Plus, (1) Green Tea Extract should be given 2 hours before or after breakfast if Shield4Pets is a part of your breakfast protocol due to the Vitamin C in the Heart Plus. If Shield4Pets is not a part of your breakfast protocol then these supplements can be added into the food mixture along with the other morning supplements.

Neutralize - approximately 30 min after Breakfast (1 to 2 tbs) Braggs Raw Organic Apple Cider Vinegar & (1tsp) raw honey, (1tsp) bee pollen diluted in warm water **– Promotes Alkalinity – Remember that cancer cannot survive in an alkaline environment.**

Early Afternoon - at least one hour before snack time – your second dose (1 tbs) of Essiac Tea should be given on an empty stomach and at least 1 hour before meals or supplements.

Snack if needed – before 4pm – the list below are a variety of options Nola ate as an afternoon snack if she was hungry.

I did not give two fruits in one snack or a fruit along with carrots due to the sugar content.

FOOD: choose from the following:

(1) raw organic carrot – all of my dogs have always loved to munch on carrots, whole, like a bone – they like the mini ones too, in place of store bought doggie treats.

(1) raw organic apple

(½) baked organic sweet potato

(1 tbs) coconut oil (Nola just licks it off of the spoon)

(½ cup) Budwigs with berries chopped up or puréed and added to the mixture

SUPPLEMENTS: not all listed have to be given at every snack, but they can be if needed:

(1) Canine Multi-vitamin

(2) Heart Plus pills (Vitamin C/Lysine/Proline/Rose Hips)

(1) Green Tea Extract (to be given along with Heart Plus to aid in efficacy of Heart Plus)

(1) Bromelain

(1) Vitamin E (Not necessary if giving a multi-vitamin at this time)

(5) fish oil pills (1000 mg each)

(5) Dried Green Barley Pills (increase over time depending on your dog's weight and tolerance – Nola gets 5 or 6 at a time for

a total of 15 to 20 a day). **Give the Dried Green Barley pills 20 minutes before the rest of the meal, which follows the dosing guideline provided by Green Supreme.**

<u>**Early Dinner Menu – between 6pm & 8pm to distance from the Artemisinin dose at 12:30am. If Artemisinin is not a part of your protocol or if it is an "off" Artemisinin dose evening, then the breakfast meal can be repeated for dinner and the time of evening is not important. Following is our EARLY dinner protocol on evenings that we DO dose the Artemisinin.**</u>

FOOD:

(1 cup to 2 cups) cooked (boiled) organic chicken breasts

(one serving) Budwigs with VERY LITTLE OR NO Greens – **I decided this depending on how close to 8pm I was feeding. If I fed Nola at 6pm then I would add greens and if I fed at 8pm then I didn't give her any greens due to their iron content affecting the efficacy of the Artemisinin.**

(½ cup) quinoa cooked

(3) fresh mushrooms chopped (any variety)

(1/2 cup) beans – any variety

(2 tbs) coconut oil

SUPPLEMENTS:

(1) Astragalus pill (500 mg) – open capsule and pour into food if desired

(5) fish oil pills (1000 mg each)

(1) D3 vitamin pill (1000 IU)

(2 tbs) ground egg shells (or 1 calcium supplement)

<u>Late Dinner Menu – 9pm or later. If Artemisinin is not a part of your protocol or if it is an "off" Artemisinin dose evening, then the breakfast meal can be repeated for dinner and the time of evening is not important. Following is our LATE dinner protocol on evenings that we DID dose the Artemisinin, but could not feed dinner until after 8pm.</u>

FOOD:

(1/4 cup) cooked (boiled) organic chicken breasts – don't feed chicken (or any meat) after 9:30pm

(3/4 cup) plain Budwigs -No greens (more can be given if needed for larger dogs)

(2 tbs) coconut oil

SUPPLEMENTS:

(5) fish oil pills (1000 mg each)

(1) D3 vitamin pill (1000 IU)

(2 tbs) ground egg shells (or 1 calcium pill supplement)

If your schedule does not allow for this much food prep and cooking time, there is a company called The Honest Kitchen, www.thehonestkitchen.com/ that has several great options for your cancer dog. I learned of this company after Nola passed and I occasionally purchase this food for my current dogs.

This is a statement taken from The Honest Kitchen website, "We believe cats and dogs deserve the highest quality healthy pet food. We provide **all natural human grade dog food and cat food products**, using dehydrated whole foods. Our pet foods are **produced in the USA from non-GMO produce, hormone-free meats and some organic, fair trade ingredients** - all carefully sourced from around the world (and we **NEVER** use any pet food ingredients from China)."

The Honest Kitchen has a product called **Kindly Base Mix**, which is grain, potato & fruit free – all you do is add water and your choice of meat. It is packed full of wonderful cancer fighting vegetables and it does have dried garlic, vitamin D3 and vitamin E in it as well.

Another option they offer, **Zeal Dog Food**, is great for cancer dogs because it is grain & potato free and full of cancer fighting ingredients as well as omega 3 from fish. Zeal has two types of dehydrated raw fish, so with this option you don't have to add anything but water, but feel free to enhance it further, if you wish.

Feeding dehydrated, raw meat and vegetables to your dog is a great way to introduce a raw diet, without a lot of effort. I trust The Honest Kitchen and feel comfortable recommending its food as a second option to fresh food preparation. The food at The Honest Kitchen has high quality, human grade ingredients and serves as an adequate base for a cancer diet. This food is somewhat expensive, especially if you have a large dog with a big appetite, so the convenience comes with a price. I have not done the math to know how the cost compares to fresh cooked meals. If you consider all the ingredients you won't have to purchase fresh, it may be comparable. Either way, this is a great back up option for those who simply don't have the extra time for the necessary food prep required in this protocol.

You can always use The Honest Kitchen food on busy days and cook fresh meals on days you have more time. Your dog will love the variety and it will feel pampered from all the extra love and attention to their meals.

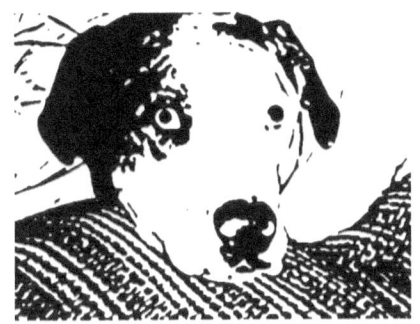

Natural Remedies for Urinary Tract Infection (UTI)

Urinary tract infections can be common for dogs with cancer for various reasons. Since we know cancer can't thrive in an alkaline environment, we work hard to create alkalinity in our pets' bodies, by giving them plenty of alkaline food & herbs. Unfortunately, pH levels that are too alkaline can cause crystals in its urine, leading to an infection and a lot of discomfort. On the other hand, cancer causes pH levels to be more acidic, when the proper food/ supplements are not given to help with alkalinity. When a pH level is too acidic, it can also cause crystals to form. A balance of alkaline and acid food is the key to a healthy pH level.

A healthy pH for a dog is between 6 and 6.5, which is slightly more acidic than a healthy pH for humans. It is very easy to check the pH with pH strips that you can pick up at any health food store, pharmacy or online.

The important thing to understand, when monitoring the pH, is certain times of day pH levels range to seem more acidic or alkaline. This is determined by mealtime, supplements, first pee in the morning and many other variables. The key is to check it several times throughout the day, if possible, and take an average. The best time to check is a couple hours before or after meals and supplements. Since it isn't always possible to get your dog to urinate when you need it to, the more you can test it, the better. I would not recommend checking its pH through its saliva, because its saliva always registers to be much more acidic than its urine because a dog's saliva is much more acid than human saliva by nature. This will not give you an accurate snapshot of what the overall pH environment looks like in your dog's body.

A more accurate option is to test pH levels with a blood test, which is very expensive. Dr. Baker explained that a blood test only takes a snapshot of the blood pH at that moment and it was not the best use of our money, when there were so many other things Nola needed at the time, with our limited funds.

I found the pH strips to do a great job of showing me how different foods affected her pH and the overall environment in her body, with regard to alkalinity, throughout the day. Of course my neighbors must have thought I was crazy, following my dog around with a pH strip and putting my hand *down there* every time she peed. Expect to get peed on a lot. It goes with the program and nothing that any parent wouldn't do for their kids, right?

Thankfully we never had to deal with UTIs during Nola's journey, but our other healthy dog, Suri, recently showed symptoms of a UTI. I immediately started her on a couple of the following remedies and her symptoms went away before it turned into anything serious. I believe Nola's diet and my regular monitoring of her pH levels helped us to dodge that bullet, while fighting cancer.

The earlier you can catch a UTI, the better your results will be to fight it naturally. **If the symptoms do not go away within a few days of natural treatments, it is important to take your dog to your vet as soon as possible.** I seldom advocate antibiotics, especially for cancer dogs, but there are times when they are necessary so your dog is not in distress and it doesn't lead to something worse. UTI's can be very serious and must be attended to immediately. They can be a sign of something else transpiring from the cancer, so it is always smart to keep your vet informed of its condition and let him or her know what you are giving your cancer warrior at all times. I kept a very detailed journal of Nola's diet. I updated it regularly and gave a copy to Dr. Baker every time it changed.

Some of the main symptoms of a UTI are frequent urination with very little success (dribbles instead of a steady stream of urine), urinating in odd places, excessive drinking, blood in the urine, fever, lethargy and excessive licking *down there*. If you have ever experienced a UTI, you know how miserable they are and these remedies will help to treat the bacteria and soothe the uncomfortable symptoms. By the way, they work for humans too. I am including my favorite natural UTI remedies below, but I have also included links that have more information on UTIs and natural remedies. All of these herbs can be purchased at your local health food store.

Juniper Berries – Juniper berries work well on even a severe UTI because they increase the rate in which the kidneys filter out impurities and increase urine production. They are safe for dogs and cats when used in moderation. You can use the berries to make a tea, which is how I use them, or you can get a certified food grade juniper berry essential oil and dilute it with water. I followed the directions for making the tea and dosing my dogs per Ottawa Valley Dog Whisperer:

(20) berries for every cup of water. Steep in a tea pot or other pot with a lid and only steep for 5 to 7 minutes to preserve the volatile oils needed from the berries. I use one to two tablespoons of tea in their food per day for no longer than four weeks, for a medium

to large size dog. Small dogs should have only one tablespoon per day.

Read more:

ottawavalleydogwhisperer.blogspot.com/2013/05/diy-natural-herbal-homeopathic_31.html

According to my *Energetics of Herbs* chart for Traditional Chinese Medicine I purchased from Dr. Baker, Juniper takes the path through the kidneys and bladder, which confirms the theory that it is a great option to cure a urinary tract infection.

Uva Ursi – According to Modern Dog Magazine by Dr. Loridawn Gordon, a naturopathic veterinarian, "Uva Ursi leaf is one of the most powerful natural astringents available. Holistic veterinarians use it to attack a variety of pathogens that are often the cause of UTIs. It can stop bleeding and reduce the inflammation associated with these infections."

Read more:

moderndogmagazine.com/blogs/loridawn/natural-relief-your-dogs-urinary-tract-infections#sthash.ZDnnSiQ4.dpuf

The article in Ottawa Valley Dog Whisperer also recommends the Uva Ursi as a good remedy for UTI. I followed their dosing recommendations, which are similar to the Juniper Berry, other than you do NOT want to use this longer than THREE DAYS at a time. Like the Juniper Berries, I used the Uva Ursi leaves to steep and make a tea. You can and <u>should</u> steep the Uva Ursi leaves longer than the Juniper Berries. Per the directions, you steep until the tea is room temperature. Read more:

ottawavalleydogwhisperer.blogspot.com/2013/05/diy-natural-herbal-homeopathic_31.html

<u>Goldenseal</u> - <u>Ottawa Valley Dog Whisperer</u> recommends Goldenseal because it is antibacterial and antifungal. According to my *Energetics of Herbs* chart for TCM, Goldenseal takes the path through the bladder and it is a cooling herb, therefore confirming that it is another great option for a UTI. You can use this in a dry herb form or tincture, so you should follow the dosage recommendations on the bottles and confirm them with your holistic vet. **Goldenseal should not be used on small puppies and kittens or pregnant or lactating dogs or cats.**

<u>Braggs Apple Cider Vinegar</u> – Is there anything that <u>ACV</u> doesn't cure? It truly is nature's wonder drug and typically my first choice for everything. You should already have this as a staple in your cancer warrior's diet to aid in alkalinity and inflammation in the body. If your pet's UTI is caused from over alkalinity, however, then you should back off of it for a couple days and try the other

remedies first. ACV has great antibacterial properties and can be used, diluted in water, to wash the exterior of the urinary tract, which is also important to keep clean during a UTI.

Cranberry or Blueberry - Quoted from Modern Dog Magazine, "Cranberry or Blueberry will prevent the bacteria from attaching to the lining of the urinary tract and is great for the prevention of recurrent infections.

Read more:

moderndogmagazine.com/blogs/loridawn/natural-relief-your-dogs-urinary-tract-infections#sthash.ZDnnSiQ4.dpuf

Parsley - Dr. Loridawn Gordon also mentions in Modern Dog Magazine, "Parsley leaf is an effective diuretic that can aid in the elimination of waste and, in addition to being highly nutritious, parsley leaves have antiseptic qualities that are great for treating urinary tract infections." Read more:

moderndogmagazine.com/blogs/loridawn/natural-relief-your-dogs-urinary-tract-infections#sthash.ZDnnSiQ4.dpuf

Like ACV, Parsley should already be a part of your cancer warrior's regular diet because it has great cancer fighting properties and it helps with alkalinity. According to my *Energetics of Herbs* chart for TCM, parsley takes the path through the bladder and kidneys, confirming that it is another great option for a UTI.

There are a lot of natural products on the market that combine several herbs, including the herbs I have listed above, as well as others that have been proven to successfully treat urinary tract infections. Since I have not used any of these products, I have chosen to not include information on them, but with a little research you can quickly find a lot of resources from which to choose. As I have mentioned before, don't fall into the trap of buying the "next best thing." When in doubt, stick to the basic ingredients. Your holistic vet should be able to recommend their favorite remedies as well. Feel free to consult with the <u>Artemisinin Yahoo Group</u> to find out what natural remedies others have used.

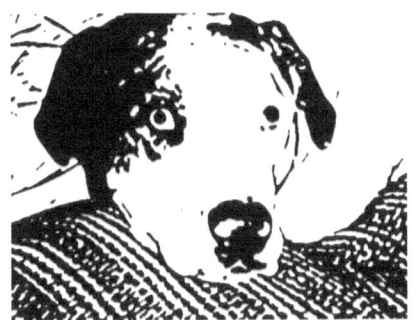

Is Amputation Right for Us?

This chapter focuses on dogs with <u>Osteosarcoma</u> (OS), which, as I mentioned, is the type of cancer Nola had. During the first visit with Nola's surgeon, he told us an interesting theory about amputating the tumor leg, especially interesting coming from a surgeon. He believes delaying the amputation of the main tumor will signal the cancer to not metastasize (spread) to other areas of the body. This is contrary to what most veterinarians or surgeons will tell you.

I wish I could tell you one theory is better than another, because I have seen equal outcomes with both theories. The other theory being immediate amputation, before the cancer has had a chance to spread, followed by a couple rounds of chemotherapy. You might be thinking, "of course the second theory makes the most sense," but let me explain a little further before you come to your conclusion. And before I do that, I want to reiterate when you are sitting in the room with this surgeon, you know you are in the presence of a genius (even though he was dressed like Jimmy Buffett) and his theory should not be taken lightly.

His theory, which was based on his many years of experience with OS amputations, is that Osteosarcoma is a very fast spreading cancer and therefore had already spread throughout Nola's body by the time we found the tumor on her leg. By keeping the main cancer source contained for as long as possible, in this case the tumor on Nola's right front leg, you are also keeping the other cancer cells dormant. Once you remove the main source, the body signals the other cancer cells to grow and metastasize. Cancer will then begin to show up in other areas very quickly.

Osteosarcoma typically spreads to the lungs and once that occurs, it is much harder to control. He explained that the tumor on her leg is never going to kill her. It's the other cancer throughout her body that will do the main damage, especially to the lungs or liver. To hold that off for as long as possible would prolong her life – in our case he seemed to be right.

Nola lived almost a year with the cancer, which are the same results that many others get that amputate immediately, followed by a couple rounds of chemotherapy. I believe there is merit to both options. I told you about Chalali, who lived approximately 2 ½ years after her OS diagnosis. Juli chose to never amputate, due to Chalali's size, and they had great success with natural medicine.

If I am faced with this decision again, I am not sure what I would do the next time, with regard to surgery. Much of my decision would depend on my dog and how well it handles pain. No matter how well you manage pain, it will experience some pain with the tumor. I feel our protocol, by the end of Nola's journey (the one that I am sharing with you in this book), was strong enough to slow and kill the other cancer cells that might have been in her body. With that regard, I would feel comfortable waiting or amputating – either way you have to fight the cancer cells, keeping them from spreading for as long as possible. A cure was never an option for us with OS, so longevity and endurance was our goal.

We spent a lot of money and energy on pain management, by postponing the surgery. The tumor slowly ate away at her bone, so pain management became as important and sometimes more important than fighting the cancer. We could have put all our efforts toward fighting the cancer, which is why I say I may choose amputation sooner, if faced with the decision again. In order to combat cancer and pain at the same time, I used a lot of natural anti-inflammatories that also fought cancer, but pain management was a huge component of our protocol because of that pesky tumor. We were lucky we had such a tough dog with a very high tolerance for pain (or just very stubborn), because she made that part pretty easy for us.

I think many dogs would not be able to handle this level of pain without a caregiver who really understands how to control it. I don't want to brag, but I was the master at pain management, to the point that Nola's leg had completely broken in half without our knowledge. The tumor was holding her leg together, so we had no idea until her last x-ray. She never let on that it was hurting very much at all. Partly because she was obviously a total badass, but I believe mostly it was because I understood the kind of pain she was feeling and had learned how to attack it from every angle. I have an entire chapter on pain management that will help with pain at all stages of cancer.

Although her pain was managed, I felt very guilty we did not realize how bad her leg had gotten. Once we knew, immediate amputation became our clear decision. After witnessing how easy it was for her to bounce back from amputation surgery and manage on three legs, we wished we had done it while she was healthier. We found out her cancer had spread to her lungs at the same visit we found out her leg was broken, so we were faced with the decision to put her down right then or amputate.

As I watched my very strong girl drag my husband down the hall at the vet's office (with a broken leg and lung mets) to chase after a cat, I knew it was not her time yet, no matter what the statistics told us. Our vet, once again, put a time stamp on Nola's life and gave her three weeks at best to live. Will he ever learn? This was still the old vet, at this time, as we chose to keep him as part of the team for regular x-rays and pain medication, since he was five minutes from our house. I have to admit, he had me very rattled and confused, but my husband and I were in total agreement, Nola was not done fighting. She was not showing any real signs of suffering at that point. Again, she was literally dragging my very strong husband down the hall after a cat. We knew we had only one choice, which was to move forward with the amputation surgery. Nola would let us know when she was done fighting and her fight was still strong.

We will never know if her cancer would have spread faster if we amputated sooner. We amputated eight months into our fight and she spent those eight months of her journey feeling pretty darn good. I realize I haven't really answered the question, "Is amputation right for us?" Unfortunately, this is a personal decision that has many variables determining what is right for you and your dog. I can only share the options we were faced with and what I would consider if faced with the decision again, God forbid. Only you know your dog and your circumstances and both options are viable. Both options show great promise as long as you focus hard, HARD, on a cancer fighting diet.

If you have a dog that is not a good candidate for amputation due to its size or age, or if you cannot afford the surgery, you should have peace of mind knowing it may work in your favor and you still have many other options. If you have a very active dog who can't handle the pain of the tumor, then amputation with chemotherapy and a strong cancer fighting diet is a good choice for your dog, because it will do very well on three legs. That part should not be a factor in your decision, unless it has other injuries or arthritis that is already hindering its ability to move around. Becoming a Tripawd is typically much harder on the humans than the dogs.

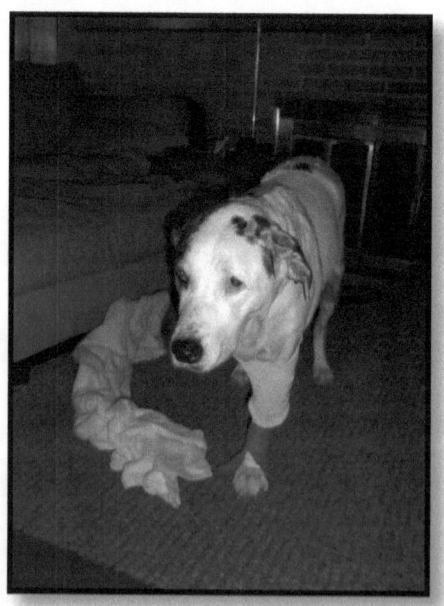

This picture was taken the day after Nola's amputation surgery. As you can see, she was able to immediately balance on three legs and get around very well. Once you join the Tripawd Yahoo Group, you will quickly learn about many success stories for this surgery.

If you choose to delay the amputation surgery, as we did, you must have a special boot made that is custom fitted to your dog's tumor leg. It will protect its leg from fractures and relieve pain when walking. This is something that you should do immediately. There are companies that specialize in this type of prosthetic. The technicians will need a mold taken of your dog's leg, which your vet can provide, and sent to them for a proper fitting. If you happen to have pet insurance, this should be covered within your plan. We did not have pet insurance and we spent $445 on Nola's boot.

We used ACE Ortho Solutions, which is the company recommended to us by our surgeon. We were very happy with their product and services. Their contact information: ACE Ortho Solutions, PO Box 471, 714 Chief St, Suite 1, Benkelman, NE 69021. (308) 423-2612. You can email Ben, the technician and main contact, at ben@ aceorthosolutions.com.

Juli used Animal Ortho Care LLC, http://www.animalorthocare. com/ for Chalali's boot and she raved about their service and product as well. After seeing pictures of Chalali's boot, I thought her boot looked more comfortable and high-tech than Nola's. Therefore, I would recommend her company every bit as much as ACE. Those are the only two companies I am familiar with, but you can and should ask your veterinarian if they recommend a company they use regularly.

Special boots for two special girls. These are pictures of Chalali (left) and Nola (right) in their custom boots. It took them a little time to get used to them, but once they did, there was no stopping them!

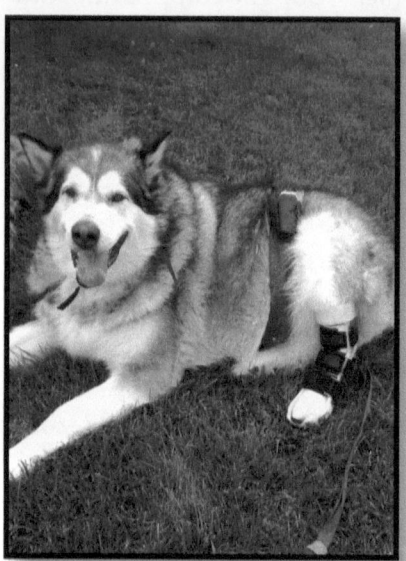 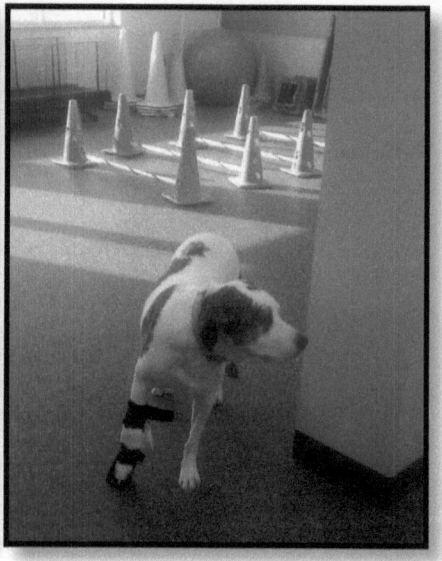

Juli said Chalali cried when she took it off, so they left her boot on most of the time. It was obviously helping a lot with pain management. We couldn't leave Nola's boot on for long periods of time without irritation from rubbing.

I hope this chapter has helped, at least a little, with this difficult decision and has not confused the issue even more. If you choose to delay the surgery, be ready to hit pain management from every angle. The next chapter will guide you through this process.

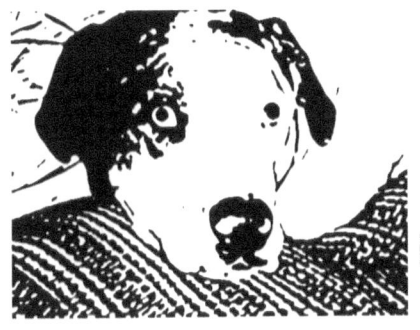

Pain Management ~ Holistic and Western Medicine work together

Rule #1, which I learned the hard way, is to treat pain full on <u>before</u> your warrior shows signs of pain. Once it feels pain, it is much harder to catch up and get back in front of the pain. I remember, in the beginning, being so proud of the small amounts of pain killers that Nola needed, so I held off giving her the full dose until it was harder to manage. I guess I felt like increasing it meant we were giving into the cancer, which meant it was winning. Once her tumor grew to a certain size, there was obviously more pain involved. I finally learned treating the pain, before she felt it, allowed her to be a very active and happy dog, with no down times. When I waited for her to show signs of pain, it took much longer to get her back to that happy place again.

With regard to narcotic pain meds, we used **Tramadol**. We were lucky Nola did very well on Tramadol. It didn't make her drowsy or other negative side effects, like panting, that some dogs experience with Tramadol. We started giving her (2) pills every eight hours, then progressed to (3) every eight hours. As we got closer to the end, we progressed to (3) every four to six hours, but that was during the last three weeks of her life.

Two to three pills every eight hours worked well for Nola for a very long time, but don't hesitate to move them closer together if you see signs of pain before the eight hours are up. You can sneak (1) pill in between doses if necessary. Dogs don't build up a tolerance to Tramadol and it can be given in pretty high doses without harming your dog, but you should always consult your vet with every dose increase. I believe the max dose for a dog Nola's size (75 - 80lbs) is (4) every four hours, but again, you will need to consult with your veterinarian for the proper dosage for your dog, depending on its size and its tolerance to the drug.

We were also given **Gabapentin** to dose along with the Tramadol when her cancer progressed toward the end, but I only gave it to her a couple times. I didn't like it because it made her really groggy and she had a hard time getting around because, at that point, she was a Tripawd (post amputation). While on Gabapentin, she stumbled and ran into furniture, so it never made it into our regular protocol. That said, many have great success with Gabapentin and it is used for nerve pain, so it works well for certain kinds of cancers, including Osteosarcoma. It's worth trying if the pain begins to affect the happiness of your warrior. Keeping them comfortable and happy should be your main goal.

That was the extent of the narcotic drugs in our pain management protocol, as I mainly relied **on <u>NSAIDS</u> (Non-steroidal anti-inflammatory drugs)** with great success. We chose all natural NSAIDS except one, **<u>Deramaxx</u>**, which Dr. Baker convinced me to continue, due to its added benefit of cancer fighting properties. I was hesitant to keep Nola on Deramaxx for a long period of time because it was so strong. She could only have ½ pill daily and I had to watch for dark stool, which would signify blood in her stool, which concerned me. It seemed to go against everything I was trying to achieve with her natural care, but we never had any issues with it and I do feel it helped a lot with our pain management. The added bonus of its cancer fighting properties helped to seal the deal for me.

When selecting natural NSAIDS, I made sure she had a wide range that attacked all areas of pain, such as broken bone pain (**Bromelain**), arthritic pain (**yucca**) and basic inflammation (**Boswellia Extract, Devil's Claw and White Willow Bark**). Since Nola died, I found a great supplement at GNC that has all of the above and more in one pill. It may seem a little pricy, but it's a fraction of the cost of purchasing all the ingredients individually. The supplement is called **<u>Dr. Joints</u>** and it has **Glucosamine, Bromelain, Boswellia, Chondroitin, Devil's Claw, MSM & Yucca**. I never used this on Nola, so I'm not sure if it would have worked as effectively as dosing the herbs individually, but it is worth a try. The salesman at GNC told me they can't keep it on their shelves because people are having great results with it for arthritic pain. I gave Dr. Joints to my mom for arthritic pain in her knees and hips and she reported back that they are working extremely well to relieve her pain. I also give it to my other aging dog, Barley, to help him when he feels stiff from playing too hard. So far it has worked well for him, but I also give him raw apple cider vinegar, turmeric, ginger and garlic, which are all great anti-inflammatory foods and are likely helping just as much.

This is a nice segue into **anti-inflammatory foods**, which are every bit as important as the supplements, if not more important. **Fresh garlic, ginger & turmeric** are the most important trio, in my opinion, and have been proven to be of the very best anti-inflammatory foods one can eat, rivaling any pain medication on the market. Plus, they are great for fighting cancer and keeping the body alkaline, which is why I make sure my healthy dogs also get this trio added into their food for cancer and arthritis prevention.

Celery, cucumber, button mushrooms and apple are also great anti-inflammatory and cooling foods, which help cool the heat condition from the cancer. And don't forget about **Raw Organic Apple Cider Vinegar** – ACV is one of nature's best anti-inflammatories and had an alkalizing effect in the body.

The next two pain management tools are options outside of pills and food. They both yield excellent results and had wonderful effects on Nola.

<u>Acupuncture</u> proved to be a powerful tool for natural pain management and surprisingly affordable. We were so lucky Dr.

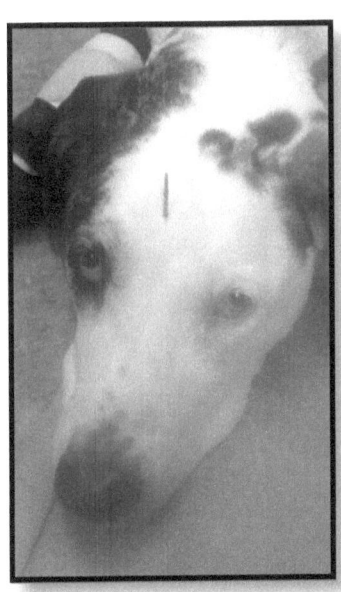

Baker was very skilled in acupuncture and offered the service within her practice. Nola responded well to Acupuncture and was noticeably pain free for several days after the procedures. This became a weekly routine as her tumor grew and Nola loved the special attention. At the very least, she loved the weekly road trip that came along with the procedure.

If you include acupuncture as part of your pain management protocol, make sure the acupuncturist is familiar with cancer tumors and they know to NOT put the needles anywhere near the tumor – you want to draw energy away from the tumor, not toward the tumor. A skilled acupuncturist will know this, but I felt it important enough to include, so you know as well. Remember, knowledge is power.

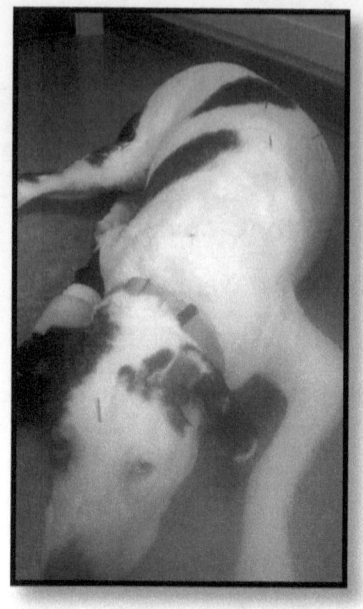

These are moments I captured with my crappy phone camera, but I think you can see how calm and relaxed Nola was during her acupuncture procedures. Believe me when I tell you, Nola did not do anything that Nola didn't like. There would be no way to get her to lie still for this treatment if she didn't love how it made her feel. The needle in her forehead was typically put in first, because it's a calming location and it really worked amazingly well.

This last picture was taken during laser treatments Dr. Baker performed on Nola's amputation wound, to help it heal faster. I believe the laser can also be used on a tumor for pain relief - don't quote me on this, but do ask your vet if this

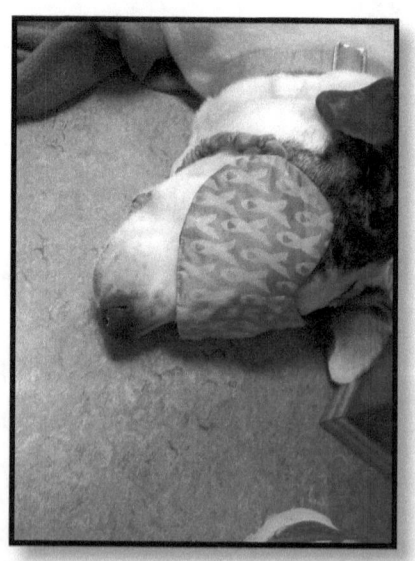

could be an option. It did not come up during our visits, but I believe that someone in the <u>Artemisinin Yahoo Group</u> mentioned this after Nola had passed. It is very easy to do, painless for the patient and very affordable. We had to wear eye protection during the laser treatment and Nola enjoyed relaxing with her eye mask – what a diva. Did I mention what a great patient she was? She loved all the attention and didn't care what we did, as long as all our focus was on her.

Last, but definitely not least, are good old **warm and cold compresses**. When Nola's tumor and pain progressed, before we had the amputation surgery, the remedy she responded to the quickest was the warm, wet towel on the tumor first, followed by a bag of frozen peas to ice it down. It gave her immediate relief. I told this to others in the Artemisinin Yahoo Group who had warriors suffering with pain from the same type of cancer tumor and some of them confirmed it was the best remedy that worked for them, for quick pain relief.

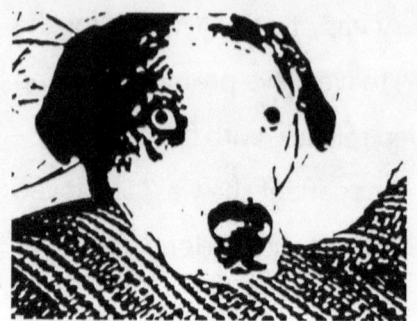

Dealing with Lung Mets

Damn, the dreaded lung mets (metastasis). The main goal for an OS warrior is to keep the cancer from spreading to the lungs. It can spread to other areas of the body as well, but the lungs are the most common place for it to metastasize first. This is why your veterinarian should be taking chest x-rays fairly often (if your warrior's cancer is Osteosarcoma) to check for lesions on the lungs. The lesions can be in the lungs for a while before your dog shows signs of them, especially if you follow my diet and feed it lots of ginger, garlic & lemon, as well as other cancer fighting foods that break up phlegm and take a path through the lungs.

I will share my favorite natural remedies to break up phlegm that you can also give your cancer free dogs when they show signs of congestion or get kennel cough. For that matter, all of these remedies work well for humans too and I use some of them all winter as I fight sinus infections and other cold symptoms.

I have re-written this next paragraph several times as I'm trying to find the right words to describe this next stage in your journey, with lung mets. I don't want you to ever give up hope, because every dog is different. I have heard of some dogs living for quite some time after the cancer metastasized to its lungs. I also need to prepare you for the reality that the lung metastasis diagnosis becomes the beginning of the end for many, as it was for us.

At this stage it becomes more about managing the cancer rather than fighting it. Until this point, you were fighting to keep the cancer cells from spreading to the lungs because, as we were told by that brilliant surgeon, the tumor on its leg won't kill it, but the lesions on its lungs or liver can. Please don't misunderstand; your fight is far from over. You still need to slow the cancer as much as possible, in hopes of keeping the lesions from taking over the lungs or from spreading anywhere else in the body.

If your warrior receives this diagnosis, there are a lot of things you can do to control congestion naturally and improve the quality of its life at this stage. You want to treat congestion the same way I told you to treat pain and that's from all angles and BEFORE it show signs.

Most remedies I will share are natural, but there is one little magic pill simply called the **cough tablet** that your vet will most likely recommend and I do too. It yields great results for keeping the phlegm loosened and the cough quiet. The main ingredients in the canine cough tablet are **<u>Guaifenesin</u> & <u>Dextromethorphan hydrobromide</u>**. The Guaifenesin is an expectorant and the Dextromethorphan hydrobromide is a cough suppressant. They are affordable and effective.

Even though I mentioned the cough tablet first, **fresh ginger** actually goes straight to the top of my list for congestion relief from phlegm, while keeping the airways free and clear. Not to mention its great cancer fighting and anti-inflammatory properties. According to Traditional Chinese Medicine (TCM), fresh ginger takes a path through the lungs (as well as pretty much every other organ in the body) and it is used to help phlegm conditions, among others. Another important TCM fact about ginger is it enhances Qi circulation, which keeps everything moving through the body, including germs and toxins, not allowing them to become stagnant.

You should add fresh ginger to its food, as part of its regular regimen, but I find ginger tea is the most effective way to use it for congestion. To make your own, steep fresh ginger (peeled & chopped) in a small amount of water with lemon & raw honey. I use this for myself a lot in the winter, when I feel a sinus infection or chest cold coming on. It immediately stops symptoms before they turn into something more serious, like bronchitis.

I give ginger tea to Suri too, for her cough. When she came to live with us, she had kennel cough, and it still tries to re-emerge every once in a while, especially in the winter. Her symptoms are very similar to my sinus infection symptoms and we both tend to get our symptoms at the same time of the season, so I can relate to how she feels and what I'm actually treating, which is mucus.

I give her two or three food syringes of the liquid from the steeped ginger, lemon & honey (ginger tea), which is all it takes to completely clear her cough. It works almost immediately, before her condition turns into full blown kennel cough. The ginger can taste pretty strong, once it's steeped, so I sweeten it with raw honey, which also soothes the throat and calms the cough. You should use a small amount of water to make it as strong as possible. I use approximately 1 ½ cups water with 1" ginger, ½ lemon with the rind & 2 heaping tablespoons of raw honey. Let it boil for a few seconds, turn off the heat and cover. Let it steep until it cools. Once it cools, you can feed it with a food syringe as well as pour some in its food. I like to use the syringe while the tea is lukewarm (not hot), then store what's left in the refrigerator, to pour over her food later.

I am excited to share with you something I just discovered today and decided to include into this chapter. I came up with a new way to administer the ginger tea, if your dog hates the food syringe as much as Suri. Nola was great with the syringe, so I didn't have this issue with her, but I really have to fight with Suri on it and I don't like to put my dogs under stress when I'm trying to help them.

Today I got the brilliant idea to mix the ginger tea into a couple scoops of canned pumpkin, which is also great for phlegm and takes a path through the lungs, according to TCM. Pumpkin also helps to sweeten the ginger tea. Don't mix in so much tea that the pumpkin becomes too soupy. The consistency of canned pumpkin makes it simple to hand feed by placing a scoop (I use my finger or a spoon to scoop and feed) onto its tongue, which it will automatically swallow when it closes its mouth – like feeding baby food to a baby and it should have the same consistency as baby food. It is full proof, you have my word. It just slides right down.

Keep this trick in mind to administer other herbs, spices or supplements, but do a taste test to make sure you don't add something that tastes gross. This is one of many great things about focusing on natural cures; you can make them taste delicious and your dog thinks it is getting pampered with special treats all day. Try to make every dose of something as pleasurable as possible. Dogs typically like the taste of pumpkin, so it can easily be used to make tasty "treats" of medicine.

I got a bit off track, but before I move onto the next remedy, I want to make sure I clearly made the point of how well ginger works – please don't discount it as a secondary treatment...**it should be first on your list**.

This next remedy should not be discounted either because it was crazy how well it worked. This was my first introduction to Essential Oils and now I'm hooked! You must use high quality, FOOD GRADE, essential oils and the only two brands I trust and recommend are doTERRA and Young Living. Dr. Baker gave the **RC Oil** (RC stands for respiratory care) by Young Living to us to try before we purchased a bottle and I honestly could not believe how well it worked.

I only used one or two drops on Nola's back foot between her outside toes. Dr. Baker instructed me to rub it in between her toes and that was all there was to it. She also stressed, ONLY ONE DROP, which I didn't understand until I used it on Suri for her kennel cough, who has a much more heightened sense of smell than Nola did. This stuff really bothers Suri for the first few minutes, but it never bothered Nola at all, so I wasn't sure why the one drop rule was so important until now.

Most dogs' sense of smell is about 10,000 times greater than ours, so if the oil is very strong smelling to us, just imagine how bad it is for them. It is important to use very small amounts and dilute it in water or coconut oil if necessary. Even though Suri is sensitive to it, I do continue to put a little between her toes when her cough flares up because it really works and it only bothers her for a couple minutes. I sometimes think it has more to do with the fact I put something on her against her will, than anything else. doTERRA has a similar oil blend called BREATHE to which I have heard others give great testimony, but I can't attest to the BREATHE oil myself. I do use doTERRA pretty much exclusively for all of my other oils, but I stick with the RC Oil from Young Living for congestion, because I know it works.

When Dr. Baker first gave it to me, I was skeptical, but willing to try anything. Every time I used it on Nola, I was shocked at how it worked on her congestion. The first couple times I wondered if it was just in my head, but over time, I couldn't deny the results because they were consistently positive.

I now use it on myself at the first sign of a cold and I love it. I open the bottle and inhale a big breath of it and rub a few drops onto my chest and the bottoms of my feet. Typically within a day my symptoms are gone. The RC Oil may seem a little expensive, but it lasts a very long time. I am still using the same bottle that I purchased from Dr. Baker over two years ago and I have a lot left. A little goes a long way with all essential oils. Other essential oils you can try for congestion are the **food grade lemon oil and wild orange** in the ginger tea and add a very small amount (one or two drops) to its food. All citrus takes a path through the lungs and breaks up phlegm, as well as aids alkalinity to fight cancer.

Once I started researching essential oils, I was enlightened and no longer surprised by their results. They've been around for hundreds of years and our ancestors used them regularly in their medical practices. Big Pharma tries to emulate the same results that essential oils have always provided naturally.

Utilizing an essential oil diffuser to diffuse the oils into the air also works well along with a **room vaporizer**, which is my next remedy recommendation. We kept a vaporizer near Nola when she was resting to keep everything moist, which helps to loosen the phlegm. Another way to do this is with a hot steamy shower. Nola always insisted on being in the bathroom when I took a shower anyway, so I let the bathroom get really steamy for her and had her stay in the bathroom for as long as possible.

Some **additional foods that help phlegm conditions**, according to TCM, are **button & shiitake mushrooms, apple peel, garlic, clam, black & white pepper, shrimp, thyme, pumpkin & watercress**. Many of these should already be in your cancer fighting diet, which is why I think Nola never showed a lot of signs of her chest congestion until the very end. Keeping inflammation down in the body and feeding these foods that take a path through the lungs and break up mucus will help every bit as much as the cough tabs because you are **treating the cause and not the symptom**. The cough tabs do a great job treating the symptom, but they will work even better when you eliminate the cause. I am aware that you can't eliminate the lung mets, once they are there, but you can minimize the amount of mucus and infection caused by the lesions with the right diet.

I remember how shocked Dr. Baker and I both were when we saw Nola's last chest x-ray, to find her lungs were completely full of lesions. I was absolutely heartbroken, but I was also very proud we were able to keep her mostly symptom free with that many lesions. At that point, she was barely coughing, and getting around pretty well without getting winded.

Milk Kefir and Budwigs are two items I have in the daily diet protocol that should be cut way back or taken out completely, once you experience lung mets. Their milky nature can make the mucus worse, so it's best to eliminate them at this time. If you need the probiotic, then you can give your warrior a probiotic in pill form to compensate.

As I have mentioned in pretty much every chapter of this book, these are great topics for the Artemisinin Yahoo Group too. I got several of these ideas, such as the steamy shower and the room vaporizer, from the group and I'm sure they have many more ideas for you to try than what I have listed. These are the remedies that worked very well for us and I am hopeful you will have just as much success with them, because they are derived from proper nutrition and the science of clean food. Understanding how these different herbs and food work and what paths they take in the body will help you to understand *why* these remedies work.

I am saying a prayer right now for your cancer warrior to have clear lung x-rays for the duration of your journey, but if that is not in God's plan, I pray these remedies work to keep your warrior comfortable and symptom free.

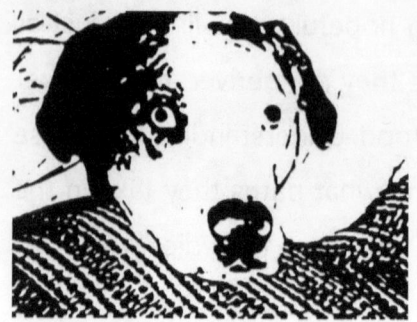

Spiritual Healing
& Meditation

If praying and meditating is not your thing, you can save yourself time from reading this section, which is why I made it its own chapter. As I explained in the beginning, the intent of this book is not to push beliefs or to persuade the reader to do exactly as we did. It is about our journey with Nola and about sharing experiences that helped us along the way.

I want to open your mind to the idea that you have many choices for healing mechanisms and they aren't all mainstream, Western medicine. I have documented what we learned and how we coped in a very difficult situation, in hopes to help you learn from our triumphs and mistakes. Prayer with meditation was at the forefront of our fight. It was in the fiber of everything we did and the guidance for every decision we made for Nola's care, so it is impossible for me to document our journey without including the experiences that fit within the topic of Spiritual Healing and Meditation.

If you choose to not read this chapter, I would like to leave you with one thought before you move on to the next. I encourage you to take time every day to sit quietly with your warrior and be in the moment with them. If you have other pets in the home let them join you; their positive energy will only help their sick companion. They know something is wrong with their brother or sister and they know better than we do how to connect on a deeper level with them.

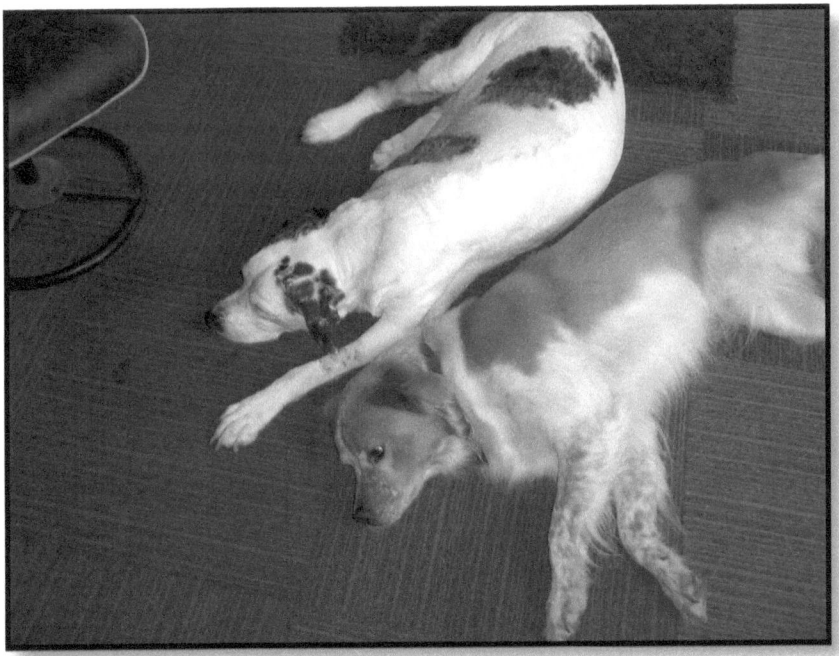

I found it fascinating that Barley spent the majority of his time watching over Nola once she became ill. Before she was ill, he never did this and they never seemed to be especially close. We rescued Barley when Nola was already a senior, so they didn't have the bonding time when they were both young. Since Barley was obviously as concerned about Nola as we were and was connecting with her in his own way, I wanted him to be a part of our healing sessions.

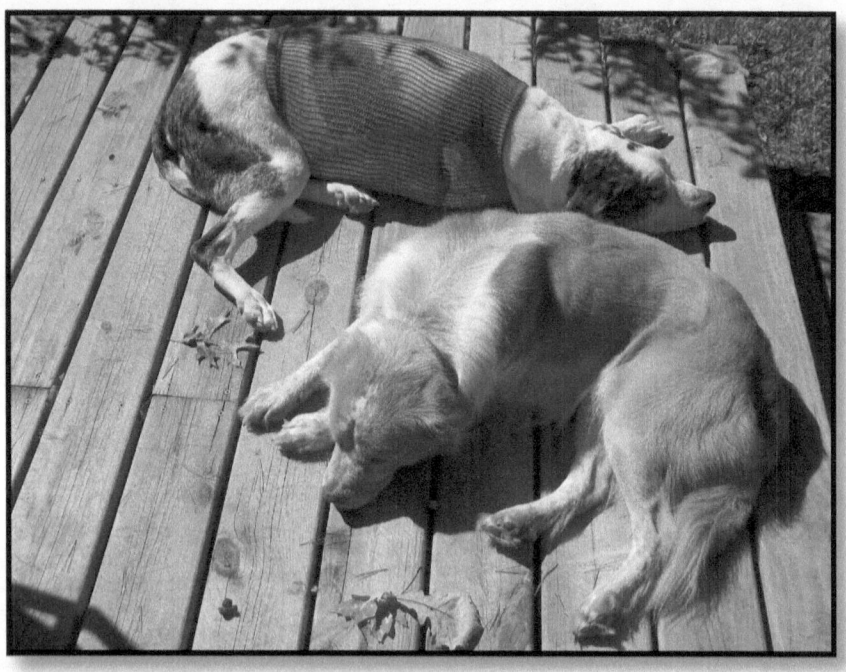

Let them know you are connecting by gently massaging and calming them with lavender essential oil, healing sounds music and softly speaking to them; however, I don't think you have to say a word because I believe they can almost read your mind, if you are tuned in enough. Sit or lie in the floor with them and let them feel your energy.

There is proof stress can cause cancer and hinder the ability to heal any disease. We all know how taxing the entire situation can be and our pets feed off of the negative energy, not to mention that stress is also detrimental to your own health. It will do you all a lot of good to take the time to *be* in the moment as often as possible. Quietly think all positive and healing thoughts.

That is what this chapter is about, only on a deeper, spiritual level.

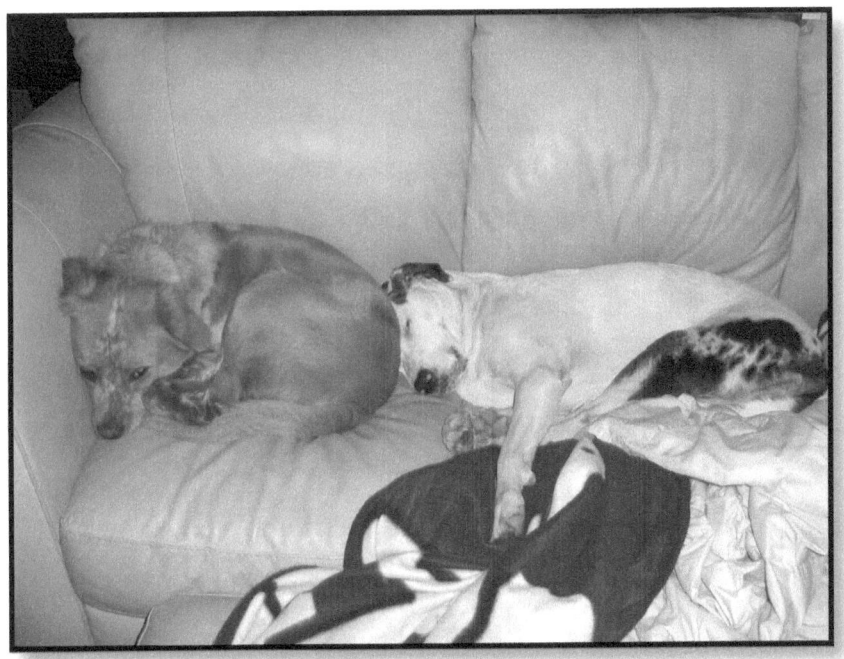

ANOINTING OF THE SICK WITH SAINT ANN'S BLESSED OIL ~ Lord God, loving Father; you bring healing to the sick through your Son Jesus Christ. Hear us, as we pray to you in faith and send us the Holy Spirit, our helper and friend. **Note:** Touch this person (dog) with Saint Ann's Blessed Oil on the forehead or, if proper, on the place of pain and pray: **Free him/her from pain and illness. Make him/her well again in body, mind and soul. I anoint you in the name of Our Lord, Jesus Christ, who lives and reigns with the Father and the Holy Spirit forever and ever. Amen** Lord God, we invoke the powerful intercession of Saint Ann. May this person (dog) be strengthened in his/her weakness. May suffering and pain be eased for your glory. May he/she be restored in total healing. You live and reign forever and ever. **Amen**

I said this prayer with Nola nearly every day, after my Catholic mother-in-law gave me a bottle of Blessed Oil from Saint Ann's Shrine, dabbing the oil on Nola's forehead, lungs and especially her tumor.

When I first started, it felt awkward and I stumbled over the words as I read them off of the card provided with the oil, which I shared verbatim, above. I would then follow with more conversations with God, asking for guidance and resources that were necessary to continue our fight. This could include crucial information and knowledge about cancer cures, availability of the necessary supplements for these cures or the resources to pay for it all.

With every day, the blessing became less awkward and I began memorizing the verses, holding onto the meaning of every word. Our prayer time grew more intense as my prayers grew stronger every day. I chose a time of day when the dogs were napping and relaxed, so I could sit with them in quiet and pray so hard that it inevitably ended in tears every time. Happy tears of rejoice, because I knew God was present and we were not alone in our fight. He was guiding my decisions and, more specifically, He was guiding my research and helping me find the information I needed in the exact moment I needed it. It was uncanny how information and resources would fall into my lap at exactly the right time. I believe if you pray with TRUE FAITH and turn it over to God, you can have peace of mind that He is in control and you can rest.

Here is an example of God at work during our journey. One day while driving, I was in deep thought about what needed to be purchased that week for Nola's care and what invoices I had out to clients that were due to be paid. I then remembered I needed to purchase her next round of Artemisinin that week, in order to get it before her current bottle ran out. I knew my husband didn't get paid until the following week and I didn't have any invoices due to be paid for a couple more weeks. Every bit of money we had in the bank at that time had to go toward food, gas and other daily living expenses, as well as Nola's pain meds, which came before all of it. I decided to turn it over to God and ask Him to help me figure out a way to make it all work because it was beyond my control. I then put it out of my mind, cranked up the radio and gave my mind a rest, knowing that God was at work.

That night, around 11:00pm, I happened to open my email within seconds of receiving an email from a guy in the Artemisinin Yahoo group who had recently lost his cancer warrior. He offered his brand new bottles of Artemisinin and Butyrex, **the EXACT supplements I needed to purchase that week**, for FREE to whomever in the group wanted them. I hated the idea of being a charity case, but I had to put my pride aside and take him up on his offer, for Nola's sake. I responded right away and explained my situation and told him about my prayer. The supplements arrived in the mail a few days later. That, my friends, is what prayer with true faith can do. I still break down in tears every time I think about that moment and how grateful I was to God for listening to me and for coming through with a solution so quickly. God's timing is always perfect. This was only one of many stories I could share with you about God at work during our journey. I honestly could write a book on that topic alone.

Another prayer that was shared with me by several friends in the dog cancer support groups is the *St. Francis of Assisi Prayer for Sick Animals:*

Heavenly Father, You created all things for your glory and made us stewards of this creature. If it is your will, restore it to health and strength.

Blessed are you, Lord God, and holy is your name forever and ever.

Amen

I am also blessed with several close spiritual friends who have strong faith in God and open minds, to explore within themselves deeper depths of spiritual connections. Each of us has different methods and motivations to connect spiritually, but we all have the same outcome, inner peace.

My friend, Heidi, has been traveling down the most interesting spiritual path through emotional healing using energy work. When Nola was sick, Heidi invited me to attend a session with her while her mentor and fellow energy worker, Penny, performed an emotional healing session on Heidi's dad before he had surgery. They did this to make sure he was fully energetically aligned with a successful surgery and recovery. Since he was out of town, Heidi acted as a surrogate for him, so I was able to witness remote energy work.

I'm not sure what happened in the room that day, but the energy was like nothing I can really put into words. It was very emotional to watch and whatever was happening to Heidi that day was also moving through all of us at the table. It surfaced specific emotions he felt at various points in his life that had remained trapped in his energy field. Then each one was released and a series of forgiveness statements, including self-forgiveness, were covered.

Afterward, Penny showed me a couple techniques to try energy work on Nola, which then became a part of our regular meditation practice. She showed me how to hold the palms of my hands very close together until I could feel the heat of my own energy between my hands. You have to really focus on it and shift into a different part of your brain to get the energy flowing – that is how it works for me anyway. You can use the energy on your dog by placing your hands over its body, very close, but not touching it. I know Nola would actually feel the heat from my hands because she would look back at the area as if I had touched her, even thought I didn't make contact with her.

To be honest, I didn't really know what to do with the energy once I found it, because I have not been properly trained, so I just did what felt right. I had watched Dr. Baker do similar things with her hands, using them to feel energy from Nola's body. I mentioned before that Dr. Baker is the best of both worlds, East and West.

I believe she was using a form of Reiki to find the areas Nola was feeling pain. I had also learned from Dr. Baker, during Nola's acupuncture sessions that you want to move the energy away from the tumor, so I did the same with the energy from my hands. I would use the energy from my palms to push energy away from her leg and tumor.

I have no idea if I was doing anything other than making myself feel better, but it was mostly about our bonding time and connecting with her on a deeper level. I plan to learn more about Reiki and other emotional release techniques someday, so I can use these practices on my healthy dogs as they age. The energy from your hands can be a great way to keep blood flowing in the joints of older dogs with arthritis...or so it would seem. I know it won't hurt to try.

The other technique Penny taught me was visualizing with light. So while I prayed and moved the energy around Nola's body, I visualized a healing light surrounding her and soaking up all of her cancer.

Now that I have *most definitely* told you all the wrong ways to use or perform the emotional release techniques, I would like to invite you to check out my friend, Heidi Straub's website (www. heidistraub.com) and learn more about her practices of Alternative and Holistic health. In addition, Heidi has agreed to share with you other resources that can help guide you in addressing the emotional component of the disease and healing journey.

A Few Words From Heidi Straub

I am very honored to have the opportunity to share with you non-invasive ways you can help your fur babies maintain their health or recover from an illness, including cancer. This section of the book is about exploring the mind-body connection. Even though it is unseen to most of us, it is just as real in animals as it is in humans. Emotional or energy healing can be one of the most powerful healing techniques you have available to you. I have discovered that almost every imbalance or illness in the body comes back to an emotional root—it starts with our thoughts and beliefs.

I have also come to learn that our pets are deeply empathic creatures. Just like we humans can literally feel and experience the emotions of those around us, pets can as well. In fact, they are often deeply energetically connected to their owners and carry much of our emotional baggage for us. As such, it is not uncommon to do energy work on pets and find that, in addition to experiencing their own trapped emotions, they are carrying a multitude of our trapped emotions. While there are a number of healing modalities that address the animals directly, it is also a good idea to clear out your own emotional baggage to prevent your fur babies from continuing to take on these energy blocks on your behalf.

As Heather has done in the rest of the book, I will attempt to expand your awareness of what is possible and point you to various resources where you can learn more. I suspect in reading through this chapter, you will find yourself drawn to one of the approaches discussed. Intuition is a very powerful thing. Listen to it and take action on it.

I want to start by building on what Heather shared above about how she worked with her body's own energy to essentially "run energy" away from Nola's tumor. You can seek out a practitioner of Quantum Touch, Reiki or another technique, but you can also supplement that work on your own. In fact, Quantum Touch is so easy to learn that you can easily begin running energy and using these healing techniques after reading the book. In addition to his book, *Quantum Touch*, Richard Gordon has certified practitioners all over the world that hold weekend training workshops.

The great news is that these forms of energy work are effective when done remotely, so you don't have to find a local practitioner in your area. If you feel called to work with a practitioner across the country, feel confident in doing so. To learn more about how to combine the power of your breath (your life force energy), your healing intent and your body's energy to heal your pet, read *Quantum Touch* by Richard Gordon or see his website at QuantumTouch.com.

For those skeptical about the ability to heal using energy alone, I encourage you to try one of the approaches I refer to as "reveal and heal" techniques. Using these techniques, you tap into the body's intelligence using muscle testing to get information about which specific emotions have become trapped in the energy field. Often times, the body will tell you that's all you need to know. Other times, you will be directed to dig deeper to find out if that emotion belonged to another person and was being empathically carried by the person or pet on which you are working. Further, you might be directed to identify the age at which it happened. Once you have revealed all the body tells you is necessary to clear the issue, you can then clear it using intention, coupled with magnets on the body's energy meridians.

Sound implausible? That was my first reaction as well. However, from my very first time of witnessing one of these "reveal and heal" techniques, I was convinced with every fiber of my being that there really is a mind-body connection. I also believe to my very core that God shows up for each and every one of these healing sessions where His presence is requested. In fact, I often "feel" the presence of Divine when I am working with clients. It is extremely rewarding when a client begins to feel the physical presence of

God with us as well, particularly when it is the first time in that person's life they have experienced that type of interaction with Divine presence on earth.

It might be useful to share a real example of circumstances that came up during one of the "reveal and heal" energy sessions I did with someone. While this example does not explicitly involve a pet, it is illustrative of the mind-body connect and our ability to carry the emotional weight for others in our lives. In addition, I have permission from the client to share this story here in the book.

A woman in her forties was experiencing extensive lower back pain, a symptom that is often associated with financial concerns or stress. I didn't know this woman's background as I'd only met her a short time before.

Through muscle testing, I was able to discern that the emotion was grief, but it wasn't her emotion. Rather, she was carrying this emotion as an empathetic response for someone else. We isolated the age to around twenty-six. Then we determined the person who was experiencing the grief at this stage in her life was a male for whom she had romantic feelings at the time.

Me: "Does this make sense to you?"

Client: "Yes."

Me: "Are you comfortable sharing more?"

Client: "I was twenty-six when I divorced by first husband. He didn't want the divorce."

(Note: Prior to that moment, I didn't know she had been previously married.)

Me: "Well, you are still carrying his grief in your energy field. I think it's time to get rid of it. First, let's see if there was a prior time in your life when you carried someone else's grief for them. Let's ask for the first time this happened to you."

After more muscle testing:

Me: "This one might be harder to believe. You were still in the womb. It was during the second trimester, sometime around the fifth month in utero, when your mom was experiencing both grief and anguish. Do you have any idea what might have happened when your mom was around five months pregnant with you that would have caused her to feel grief and anguish?"

Client: "Oh my goodness. When my mother was five months pregnant with me, her father died unexpectedly."

In the dialog that followed, the client shared that her parents had moved in with her grandparents when they found out they were going to be having a baby. The grandfather had just purchased a new, larger home that would accommodate a growing, multi-generational family. Since her grandfather was an entrepreneur and the primary contributor to the family's income, his passing created a great deal of financial concern and anxiety for the entire family. From this session, we came to realize that even the unborn child was picking up on these emotions.

As this client's story illustrates, the mind-body connection often happens on the subconscious level. The root of what is causing an imbalance in the energy field may not even be something for which the client has a conscious memory. Regardless, by tapping into the body's innate intelligence, we can surface and release these trapped emotions or disharmonious energies and clear the way for self-healing.

Interested in learning more? Of course, it is always helpful to work with experienced practitioners as you are getting started. For those of you wanting to learn to apply one of the "reveal and heal" techniques on your own, I recommend the book *The Emotion Code* by Dr. Bradley Nelson. It is a very easy-to-read book and can be applied immediately. You can use *The Emotion Code* at home to supplement any work you are doing with trained practitioners. The more trapped emotions and imbalances you address energetically in the body, the faster the body heals.

In addition to *The Emotion Code*, I also use another system that was created by Dr. Bradley Nelson called *The Body Code*. It encompasses *The Emotion Code*, as well as a fairly comprehensive set of other imbalances that can be underpinning your dog's health issues. *The Body Code* is not as straight forward to learn at home and is far more expensive to purchase, so I recommend you work with a Body Code practitioner.

In the Body Code, you can identify and address imbalances in organs and the skeletal system. You can also surface issues with nutrient deficiencies or foods that are causing irritation or reactions. Using applied kinesology (simple muscle response testing), you are able to quickly and easily tap into the innate intelligence of the body, remove the blocks and allow the body to heal itself. While these tools are designed for use with people, they work equally well on animals of all types.

To learn more about *The Emotion Code* or *Body Code*, visit healerslibrary.com.

Of course, you are welcome to reach out to me as well. I would be happy to help point you in the direction I believe is most appropriate for your needs.

In summary, I encourage you to embrace the power of your intent to heal and the profound self-healing available to all of us—animals and humans alike. Our bodies have tremendous power to heal ourselves, yet it can only be achieved in relaxation response. As you know, in this modern society, most of us live in non-stop stress response. As such, it is critically important to follow Heather's recommendations above to initiate a regular practice of prayer, mediation or yoga. This recommendation is backed by science and is explained more in the documentary The Connection — a film that explores the mind-body connection and the science behind it.

I wish you the best of luck in your journey with your brave dog. I believe the concepts and knowledge you are gaining from this book will create a foundation on which you will improve the health of everyone living in your home. I pray that God guides you and provides you with a clear knowing about the approaches that are right for you and your family. I look forward to hearing all the success stories from people who have benefitted from the knowledge Heather is gifting to the world by documenting their journey in an effort to make it that much easier for others. Love and Light to you.

Heidi Straub

www.heidistraub.com

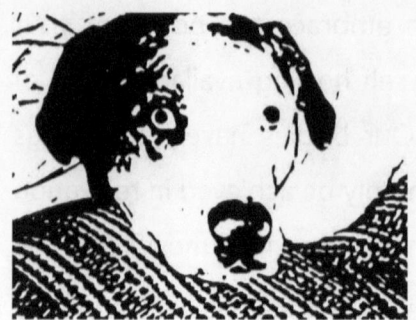

How will I Know When it's Time?

This question will be in the back of your mind the entire duration of your journey. The expenses start to compile, as well as the amount of research needed to stay in front of this disease and you wonder continuously, "How much is too much?" As long as you know you have a chance, you will do whatever it takes and NOTHING is ever too much, but you battle with the question of whether you are doing it for selfish reasons and whether your warrior is suffering.

All of these feelings are completely natural and everyone experiences them. If you have not taken my advice yet and joined the Yahoo canine cancer groups then stop what you are doing and do yourself this one favor. I can't say enough about how these groups help with these tough decisions along the way. There is always someone in the group either going through exactly what you are going through at the time or they have experienced it in the past. You will begin to see similar signs occur in other dogs just before they cross the rainbow bridge that will help you to recognize them if/when your dog begins to decline. On a better note, it will also help you to recognize the signs of issues that come up along the way that aren't serious and are easily treatable, putting your mind at ease. It isn't possible to include, in this book, every little issue that could come up during your journey. My biggest service to you is to convince you to join the groups. I want you to have the ongoing support and knowledge, at any hour of the day, from fellow dog cancer warriors all around the world.

Everyone's journey in this fight takes a different path; some are really long, windy roads and some are short cuts to the same destination. The reality is none of our pets, healthy or sick, live long enough and as they age we are always wondering the same question, "How will we know when it's time?" For us, the decision at the end was pretty dramatic and a little unexpected. It was becoming painfully clear something had changed in my beautiful, strong girl and her body was beginning to fail her. We were at the point in our journey when we knew we were no longer fighting cancer, rather just keeping her as comfortable and symptom free as possible, until our remedies stopped working.

I was pretty diligent on staying in front of symptoms the entire time we fought her cancer and I believe this is why she was never in much pain. I treated the congestion and phlegm management, once Nola had lung mets, the same as I did the pain management, when we were dealing with her tumor. When I say I was diligent, I mean Nola had around the clock care, to make sure I dosed everything at the correct times to treat pain and congestion, before she showed signs of them. I am only mentioning this again because it was easy to make the decision to let her go, once everything that was working before stopped working. I could no longer keep her comfortable, no matter how hard I tried. I was able to keep her from the dreaded coughing until the last couple days, but we did reach a point where nothing was helping. She started showing all of the signs that we knew were only going to get worse. Her medicine (both natural and western) stopped working.

She also started losing control of her back legs, which I have heard others in the Artemisinin Yahoo group mention. Her hind legs started knuckling over when she walked and this took her situation from manageable to suffering, almost over-night. At that point, I knew the end was near and made the dreaded appointment with Dr. Baker for the following week, to make sure we had her on the schedule in case we needed it. It was very important to me that Dr. Baker be the one who helped her cross, since she was there with us through the entire journey and was so wonderful to our girl. That night I had to call and bump the appointment up to the following morning. That was the part I had mentioned was very dramatic.

I will be the first to admit I pretty much snapped in that moment and I was trying so hard to hold it together for my girl. Nola was one of those dogs that understood every word I said. I wanted her last night at home to be peaceful and happy and her last night with her mommy to be special - not with me completely freaking out. So I sucked it up and made up my mind to be strong for my girl and to keep my promise.

From the beginning, I promised her as long as she was strong enough to fight and wanted to fight, I would be right there fighting alongside her. But as soon as she was no longer happy and comfortable and could no longer fight, I would help her cross. I vowed I would not keep her around due to my own weakness of not being able to let her go. It was the hardest thing I have ever done, but it was the greatest gift I could give her. I wanted her to go out with dignity. My girl was the most self confident dog I have ever known and I didn't want her to lose that confidence. I chose to maintain her dignity and let her go with very little suffering.

There is a sweet spot between managing symptoms and still enjoying life and realizing the pain has increased beyond a comfortable zone to only get worse. I feel we let Nola go in the perfect sweet spot, before things got really bad. Letting her suffer was never an option.

Your pet's symptoms are going to be different than Nola's, depending on the type of cancer and the willpower of your dog. Some dogs can't handle pain and it will show it very early on. That doesn't mean it's weak, it just means its body is more sensitive to pain. That also doesn't mean it's time to help it cross, but you do need to get in front of the pain or your dog will suffer and will not be able to sustain the endurance it needs for this journey.

You must listen to your dog because it really will tell you when it's time. When it no longer wants to do the things that would typically make it joyful and excited - pay attention. That is when you have to evaluate how much its disease has progressed and decide if you are at the point of fighting or managing. As long as you are fighting and it seems to be up for the fight, then don't stop. When you know there is nothing more you can do and it is suffering, you need to help it cross. You don't want it to suffer unnecessarily, in my opinion. Everyone says, "You will just know" and you will. No one else has the connection you have with your pet, so listen to your warrior and let it tell you what it needs. Letting go is hard, but not nearly as hard as watching it suffer.

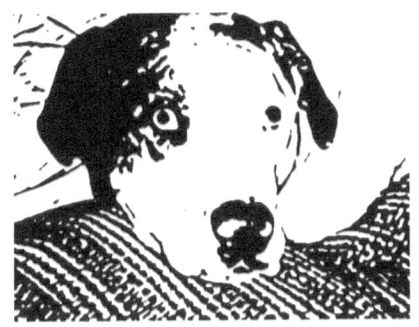

New Discoveries since our Journey

Today is February 4, World Cancer Day. How appropriate I am sitting down to write a chapter on new discoveries for cancer cures on World Cancer Day. I love it when the stars align.

Since Nola passed, I have learned about a few new cancer fighting remedies I think are worthy of sharing, even though I did not get a chance to try them on Nola. That is what I mean by "buying time." We didn't have enough time to learn about and try everything. It makes me very happy to think we may be able to buy that time for the next warrior, by sharing our information.

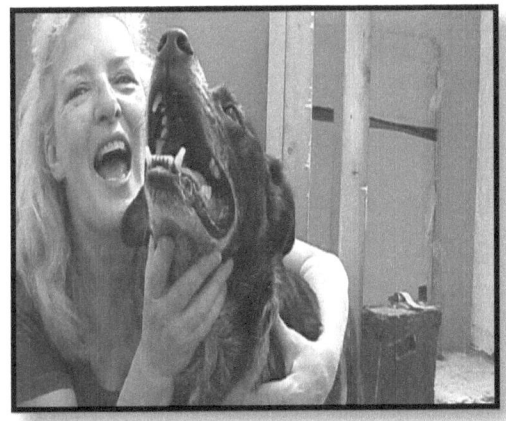

I learned about the mind blowing results for **Castor Oil** just a few days after Nola died. Yes, plain old castor oil. It was a bittersweet moment when I met

Anita & Charlie, shown here, and not to be confused with Ellen's Charley, who I mentioned earlier. Anita is a brilliant Australian who believes in natural cures and is fighting Charlie's cancer by putting castor oil on the tumor and letting Charlie lick it off. Anita also feeds him (present tense because Charlie is still blowing the vets' minds after two years) a healthy cancer fighting diet with other natural remedies that she happily shares with the <u>Artemisinin Yahoo Group</u>. I have been following Anita & Charlie's progress with the castor oil treatments through their entire journey and it has been fascinating to watch. Hopefully Anita will write a book someday and tell their story, because it's a truly incredible journey and worthy of serious consideration. Their story is way too long for me to go into details in this chapter, but you can connect with Anita in the <u>Artemisinin Yahoo Group</u> and ask her anything you want – she is happy to help.

I have to share with you the email I just received today from Anita, which Anita emailed out to the <u>Artemisinin Yahoo Group</u>. Again, how ironic (or meant to be) she sent the email on the very day I am sitting down to write this chapter ABOUT THEM! The stars are definitely aligning for me today. Following is Anita's email with her fantastic news:

```
"I'm so excited. My whole being is
brimming with elation! It's now been
2 years since I found a lump growing
```

on Charlie's leg. It's been 19 months since the vet cut it out (no clear margins) and 16 months since it grew back again and so I took him back and the vet said 'I'm sorry, I can't help him. More growths will happen in a short space of time, all over his body, and all over his internal organs'. So I took him to another vet who said the same thing.

Today I plucked up my courage and took him back. I must say the vet was very surprised to see us. I wanted to see if Charlie had any other growths that I couldn't see. Internal ones. But NOTHING! His heart is great, teeth, coat, lungs, an absolute clean bill of health. He watched him walk and noted that there wasn't a limp. He said the growth on his rib cage was a non-malignant tumor, and a couple of other little ones were just fatty growths. He asked me what I was giving him, and just said to keep it up, obviously it was working. He was even surprised that the smelly growth on his leg hadn't got any bigger, and felt it, and that was it. He also surprised that Charlie had survived eating blood and bone, which is very toxic.

I may sound like I'm skiting after all the bad news here recently, but

I thought I should spread my elation around. Better than bad news eh. Anyway, if anyone wants to know my secrets, I'm happy to tell. I've done lots of research on the net. They will sound silly and stupid and basic, but I'm of the belief that a dog knows what he has to eat when he is sick, and even though we might not think they are tasty, dogs know. At least Charlie knows.

Onward we march

Anita and Charlie (my love)"

When I read Anita's emails, I do so with an Australian accent in my head, so no matter what she says it's going to sound awesome, but this email made me so excited I could barely contain myself. I love success stories like theirs – beating all odds. This is also a great example that supports my earlier point about connecting with these groups; you are connecting with people all over the world who are sharing very valuable information. I am so thankful to have met Anita & Charlie and feel honored to have been invited into their lives to watch their very successful journey of fighting cancer naturally, with castor oil of all things.

I was getting ready to move on to my next new discovery when I saw a new email come in from Anita, sharing her protocol with the group. It is short and sweet and packed full of key ingredients. Following is the protocol, copied straight from Anita's email. Don't forget to read it with an Australian accent.

"I'll post Charlie's diet here. It seems a few people are interested, so here's the stuff.

Every morning he gets cooked chicken necks with veges and a quarter teaspoon of tumeric. Every night he gets either a teaspoon of castor oil, or a mix of a teaspoon each of bicarb soda and coconut oil. He has special patches of grass that he hoes into. I used to make him keep walking, but now I just watch him eat. Sometimes he's not interested, but most of the time he munches for about 10 minutes. His appetite is great, and every now and again I give him a couple of drops of hemp oil which someone gave me. That's about it. No tablets, no medications.

He never vomits after eating the grass, so it seems to me it's part of his diet. When he ate blood and bone he ate a different grass which made him vomit, and the next day he was fine. I originally went through a bottle of artemisinin, but because of the cost I didn't keep going after that. However I have every faith that wormwood in a pill is a good fighter of cancer and would say nothing bad about it.

He also gets apple cider vinegar - a dash - every day in another meal. He eats 3 meals a day. I'm sorry I can't tell you what the cancer is called, but it's not an osteo. Apparently it's one you see on horses. I've been told the name and forgotten, but there is a picture of it attached. It's about 3 inches round and changes all the time. One of the big bobbles disappeared about two months after this was taken. I sure hope this helps another darling. And even if you don't believe me, and are a believer of modern medicine, taking any of Charlie's remedies is NEVER going to hurt your pet, or stuff up their kidneys.

Love to you all and your dogs

Anita and Charlie (my love)"

Thanks for sharing Anita! I'm praying for you and Charlie, the cancer warrior, ever day as well as all the other badass cancer warriors out there!

Before moving on, I decided to do a little research on Castor Oil to see if I could find more evidence and studies on fighting cancer with castor oil to share with you. I found some helpful information written by Dr. Mercola on <u>Mercola.com</u>. The main points he shared, that stood out to me as very helpful for fighting cancer, are the following:

1. Castor oil has been found to have a strong suppressive effect on some tumors.
2. Castor oil boosts the lymphatic system, which supports the immune system.
3. Castor oil is an anti-inflammatory – which is vital for fighting cancer.
4. BE CAUTIOUS to not over-do it as it can give your dog diarrhea or a belly ache. (You will notice that Anita only gives Charlie a small amount daily.)
5. BE CAUTIOUS about what brand of castor oil you purchase because much of what you find in the store is made from seeds that have been sprayed heavily with pesticides.

Read more:

<u>http://articles.mercola.com/sites/articles/archive/2012/04/28/castor-oil-to-treat-health-conditions.aspx</u>

The next remedy is another gift from Mother Nature that sushi lovers will be excited about. It is the cancer killing effects of **wasabi**. I'm talking about *real* Japanese wasabi, not the green paste you typically get with your sushi rolls. I confess I didn't know there was a difference until I looked it up and read <u>the following by Dr. Andrew Weil</u>, " First of all, you should know that the green paste that usually comes with sushi isn't really wasabi. It is a combination of horseradish, Chinese mustard and green food coloring...The ubiquitous bright-green paste that you are familiar with will make your eyes water and can clear your sinuses, but it has no significant health benefits, and much of it is artificially colored." Real wasabi is a different story..."

Read more:

<u>http://www.drweil.com/drw/u/QAA400594/Wondering-About-Wasabi.html</u>

Upon further research I found an article called, *How Wasabia japonica kills cancer*, where they give more science behind the theory and explain how it works. Here is a small piece of the article to give you the basics, but the article goes into much more detail, "Scientific researchers already knew that a chemical found in *Wasabia japonica* and to lesser extent in other related vegetables, called Isothiocyanate, appeared to stop the growth of cancer by causing apoptosis, or cell death, in cancer cells. But researchers didn't know why, and because they didn't know how, science was unable to confirm that *Wasabia japonica* killed cancer cells.

Now though, <u>recent research at Georgetown University</u> found that these vegetable Isothiocyanates sticks to a defective protein found in cancerous cells through the tubulin. The Isothiocyanate chemical only binds to the protein when it is defective, and the protein is only defective when the cell is cancerous. The normal protein and cell are left alone." Read more: <u>https://wasabi.org/articles/medical-uses-of-wasabia-japonica/ how-wasabia-japonica-kills-cancer/</u>

I was first informed of the effects of wasabi in the following email from Peggy in the <u>Artemisinin Yahoo Group</u>, where she shares a discovery that wasabi can be used in place of Tumexal, that is supposed to have positive results for shrinking cancer tumors. When I researched Tumexal during our journey, I found that it was way out of our budget – very expensive – and I heard both positive and negative results from those in the group who were using Tumexal. It worked great for some and didn't work at all for others. To be able to try wasabi in place of Tumexal is exciting and well worth trying. It certainly isn't going to hurt anything. I would try Dr. Weil's recommendation of using capsules of freeze-dried genuine wasabi extract that you can pick up at your local health food store.

Following is Peggy's email where she shares the dosing recommendation:

> "Hi All Just heard about Wasabi 1 tsp a day does the same thing as tumexal...... it enables the P53 gene to kill the cancer cells......Of course only cancers that respond to the P53 gene work. I think when I finish tumexal, I will switch to wasabi....plus arte and essaic tea....Xray again in 2 weeks.
>
> Peggy
>
> Ps. can not give rymydal with wasabi or tumexal"

Olive Leaf Extract is one of my latest discoveries that I stumbled upon on the internet. I already knew olive oil is a great addition to a cancer fighting diet, because of the compound oleuropein, which is responsible for most of olive oil's health benefits. What I did not know is that olive leaves contain high amounts of oleuropein, which makes their extracts more potent than just adding olive oil to the diet. I would do both if I had to do it again. Oleuropein is also great for preventing cancer, so add it to your healthy pets' food too.

Following is a paragraph from the article on RealFarmacy.com, from which this information was found, that I found especially encouraging. "As mentioned, because oleuropein enhances antioxidant activity throughout the body it's a potent cancer preventative. Olive leaf extract protects cells from DNA damage due to oxidative stress, which is how malignant cells initially proliferate. It also disrupts the chemical signaling pathways that tumors rely on to organize, as well as inhibiting tumor growth factors. Interestingly, in one recent study, animals with tumors were given oleuropein and within 9 to 12 days the tumors were gone! [4]." Read more:

http://www.realfarmacy.com/simple-leaf-prevents-stroke-hypertension-diabetes-alzheimers-more/

That's all I have thus far, for new remedies that have excited me since Nola passed. I hope you have great results if you try them – feel free to reach out to me and let me know if you do!

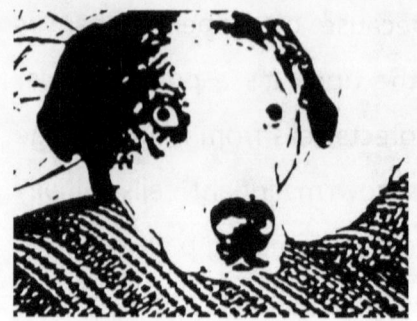

Coping with the Loss of Your Beloved Pet

I hesitated to include this chapter because I want this to be a positive book about choices that empower the reader. I then decided I have to include it because this book is also about our journey with Nola. Losing her and learning to live without her was part of that journey. Coping with her loss was very hard for me and I feel I would not be doing the reader justice if I did not share the coping mechanisms that really helped me to move through the dark, grieving period into a life where I can now remember my girl with a smile...most of the time. There are still a lot of tears, especially while writing this chapter, but they are typically followed by a smile because I'm so happy I have those memories to cherish. Dr. Seuss said it best, "Don't cry because it's over, smile because it happened."

I feel so blessed to have had the opportunity to love and enjoy such a brilliant and beautiful creature as Nola Diers. I am honored to have had the title of Nola's mommy and caregiver. She has changed my perspective on life forever and for that I am grateful.

I also feel this topic is important because it's inevitable, at some point, we will all lose our pets, even if just from old age. It's just as devastating, no matter when or why they pass. Having coping mechanisms can help you manage the grief from the loss and help you to move on to a life without them.

I don't want you to read this chapter until you need to. Your fight is not over, so don't start planning for the worst. Be positive and know only God knows what is going to happen along your journey. Your cancer warrior is only worried about being happy in this moment. Focus on keeping it happy, right up until the end. At this point, I am asking you to stop reading this chapter and to start fighting. When and ONLY when it is time to let it go, whether it's from cancer or simply old age, I invite you back to join me in the rest of our journey. I will share with you my coping mechanisms and what to expect after your warrior crosses the rainbow bridge.

I would love to welcome you back, but I know the circumstances that brought you here and I know the emptiness you are feeling. There is no point in sugar coating it -it is beyond devastating, it sucks and there is really no other way to describe it. Please know that you are not alone – you feel alone, but you really aren't. I've been there and so have millions of other pet owners out there that have loved their pets like children and have grieved their deaths the same. We understand. We get it. Many won't - forget them. Don't give them another minute of your time.

This is *your* time to grieve and to make sense of the horrific experience you just had and it's okay to feel every emotion you need to feel to get through it. You have to walk through the darkness and absorb it before you can reach the light. Don't be ashamed of feeling this way over an animal. People who feel these precious souls aren't worthy of our grief and feel we shouldn't grieve as much as when losing a human are ignorant and wrong. As you can see, I don't mince my words on this topic and I'm not afraid of offending anyone over it. I have seen "non-animal friendly" people insult animal lovers with heartless comments countless times, without caring, so why should I?

The empty space of time was the first thing that caught me off guard. As Nola's primary caregiver, I didn't consider what it might feel like when the fight was over and there was no more researching, logging meals, tracking supplements, monitoring pain - the list is endless. Every moment in time was accounted for and it was all related to her care. Everything else in life came second. All of a sudden, *poof* it's over. Your life as you knew it just stops. No more alarms throughout the day, alerting you to give the next dose of something. No more excuses to friends of why you can't go anywhere that would take you out of the house longer than four hours. And no more worry. Over, just like that. It becomes an empty space of time that needs to be filled, but with what? Grief? Sulking and feeling sorry for yourself? Crying? Yes, actually, it *will* be filled with all of those things for a while and that's okay.

Your emotions are raw and vulnerable and you need to understand them and let them out. You need to cry, A LOT. Crying is therapeutic and may seem like it takes you to a darker place, but think of crying as a lifeline that has you by the hand and is running with you, pulling you toward the light. That is what crying does, as well as laughing. The two together will heal your soul faster than any drug you can take to hide it. For a while I wasn't sure I would ever stop crying.

When Nola got to the point that I had to give her pain medication every few hours, I started taking her to work with me on the days I watched my mom's art gallery. Of course, Nola loved the extra attention and our customers became as invested in her story and her fight as everyone else who knew her. So you can imagine

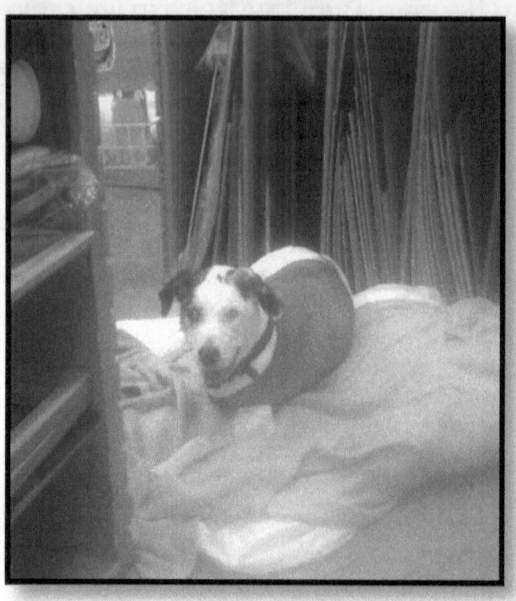

how many customers I stood with and cried, over and over, as they learned of her passing.

I also found myself feeling extra emotional over tiny things I normally wouldn't have cared about. My empathy meter was on high alert and I empathized and cried with someone over something at least once a day – that was in public. In private, I was a complete mess. Other than the two days a week I work in the gallery, I work from home, which was great as Nola's caregiver, but after she passed it was a constant reminder of where I spent all of my time caring for her. So for a while, I was crying most days, more than not crying, and this went on for about a month.

A month doesn't sound like much time to me now, but when you are crying all day, every day, a month feels like an eternity. Then one day I woke up and I was all cried out – that's when I began to see the light again. My mood felt lifted. Don't get me wrong, the crying went on much longer. Well, at this point Nola has been gone for two years and I still have moments that will send a tear down my cheek, but now they are accompanied with a smile. I actually force myself to *feel* her and remember her as often as possible. I don't ever want to forget how it feels to miss her. I want her to know that her life and death have meaning and I want to *always* miss her. If pain comes along with missing her, then I'll deal with it, because missing her keeps me connected to her.

You can only fill the empty space of time with tears and grief for so long before full on depression sets in, so give yourself time to be sad, but not too much time. Your goal is to move through the darkness, not stand still in it. In the same way that prayer with meditation was at the forefront of our fight during our journey with Nola - as I mentioned in the chapter, *Spiritual Healing & Meditation* - it was also the main thing that got me through the darkness after she was gone.

I continued to fill some of the empty space of time connecting with our other dog, Barley, who was also missing Nola very much. I connected with both of them during meditation time when Nola was sick and I didn't want Barley to miss out on special bonding to heal his heart, now that she was gone. This included quiet time together while connecting with each other through petting, massaging, kissing, nuzzling and just *being* together, while praying and meditating. I still do this often with both my current dogs, Suri and Barley. I sometimes talk to Nola during this time and sometimes to my dad who passed in 2007 and who was also a crazy animal lover. I ask him to watch over my girl until I can be with them both again and to keep her in line because I know she is up to no good, somewhere in heaven. She's probably bossing the angels around as we speak. I have no doubt my dad and Nola are together. To think this way brings me peace. If you think I'm being silly, that's fine. I don't mind, because I know what I know and I know that they are together. I don't really care what anybody else thinks, or what they think of me, for that matter. And *you* shouldn't either.

As crazy as the next suggestion may sound (or not), there are support groups with other pet owners who have recently lost their beloved children with fur and they are feeling the exact same way you are feeling. Your friends and family are there for you, but only people feeling the same darkness truly know how you are feeling right now and I think it is a great idea to seek out these groups if you feel the need to talk. I learned of one that was being held at Dr. Baker's practice, <u>Bargersville Veterinary Hospital & Wellness Center</u>, and I signed up without thinking twice. I never ended up attending it because it was a month away from Nola's passing and I had already spent a month in total darkness, reliving the experience in my head over and over. By the time the meeting was held, I was starting to get to a good place, as I mentioned before, and didn't want to move backwards into the darkness by reliving it all over again. If the meeting had been held right after she passed, though, you better believe I would have been there.

It helps to talk to fellow animal lovers who have grieved the loss of their pets, because they come with great advice. This is another important reason to join the <u>Artemisinin Yahoo Group</u>. If you already have, then you are already feeling the love and support from the group. They are probably better than a live support group because they *hopefully* have been there with you throughout your journey and they continue to be there at any time of the day you need them. They all know you and share your pain, which is what any support group is about.

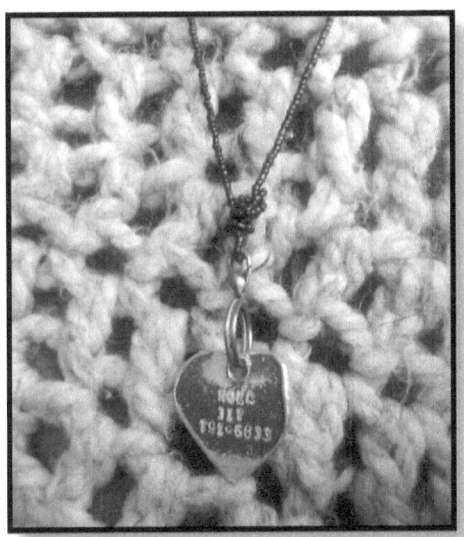

I hold the next suggestion close to my heart, literally. We had Nola cremated and they sent her home to us with a pamphlet that included advice on how to cope after the loss of your pet. In my opinion, the best piece of advice they gave me was to take a tag from

Nola's collar and put it on a keychain, to honor and remember her. I loved this idea so much that I decided to put Nola's tag on a necklace and wear it close to my heart. I have not taken it off since, other than to shower or if I'm going to an event, like a concert, where I would risk losing it, to never find it again. I sleep in it and wear it every single day. The second I put her tag around my neck, my tears started to dry up. Every time I felt the urge to cry, I would hold onto her tag and it made me feel close to her. It still does and I still have those moments.

The tag I chose is the heart shaped tag my sister, Sandi, had made for her as a gift, when she was a puppy, with her name and phone number. Nola wore it her entire life, so it is worn out and faded and I personally think it makes a fabulous fashion statement. Oddly enough, it goes with almost everything – in my eyes. I used a removable clasp so I can easily wear it on different chains, hook it onto a bracelet, or just slip it into my pocket. I mostly wear it close to my heart. This beautiful little lopsided tag was worn away from time and perfectly imperfect, just as she was. It is the most valuable piece of jewelry I own. Everything else can be replaced, but her heart will never be replaced and my necklace is a reminder of that every day. There is no amount of money that could match its worth to me, which is the same way I feel about my girl.

If you don't have a tag, you can also have necklaces made with a locket of their ashes or an imprint of their paw, which I still plan to do someday since Dr. Baker was kind enough to have an impression of Nola's paw made, as a gift, before she was cremated.

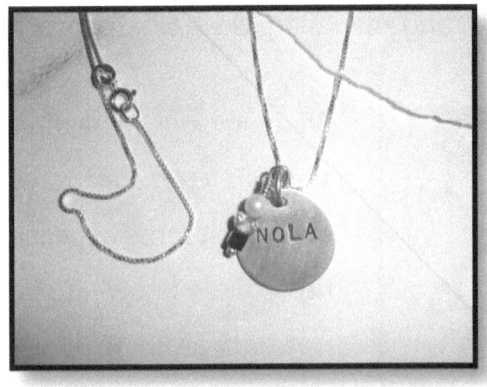

I have two other necklaces that honor Nola. One necklace has Nola's name engraved, which was made by my friend, Stacey Cassell, who is a jewelry artisan and fellow animal lover. It came as a surprise package in the mail after Nola died. I was so touched that she would take the time to honor Nola in such a special way. Stacey's necklace is a great replacement for me when I have to dress nice and the dog tag just doesn't cut it. Those are the days I slip the tag into my pocket and wear this beautiful work of art.

I purchased the last necklace from the <u>Tripawds' Etsy shop</u>. The three hearts on the front and three tiny paws on the back represent Nola's last stage in life as a Tripawd. As you can see in the picture, I also included her date of birth and death on the back. I'm sharing these to show you there are many options for keepsakes that will help you to honor your warrior and keep them close to your heart.

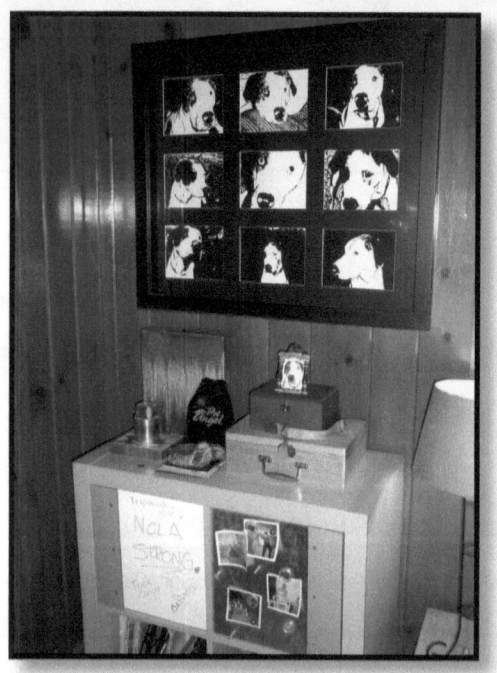

Bringing Nola home after she was cremated gave me a great sense of peace right away. Knowing she was back at home where she belonged felt right. We have her shrine in one of the main areas of our family room where she is still a focal point in our lives. It includes a collage of photos of her on the wall above her ashes, letters she received from friends in the Arte group, cards from my loved ones, her collar, her footprint and a painting of her that my mom painted years ago. They are all out for me to easily access, whenever I feel like holding them and saying a prayer for her and all of the other cancer warriors out there. This is a picture of Nola's little corner in our home where she will remain as long as we live here. Her ashes are in the small wooden box that has her collar wrapped around it and her picture on top. I created the black and whites years ago, when Nola was young and healthy, and they already hung in this location. It seemed like the perfect place to create her shrine, where she will forever rest in peace.

There are many other ways you can honor your warrior that will keep their loving spirit alive and give them the respect they deserve. On May 4, 2014, which would have been Nola's 12th birthday, we planted a gorgeous pink lilac bush by our mailbox in memory of our special girl. Now I get to think of her every time I pull into my driveway.

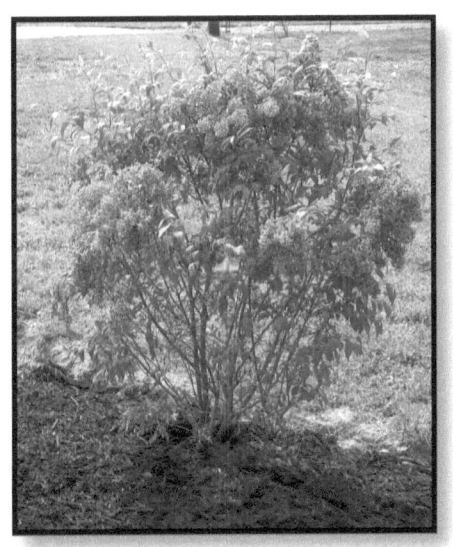

This bush is in full bloom every year on her birthday, so I also get to pick a beautiful birthday bouquet of lilacs to place by her ashes, to honor her special day.

All of these little things were helping me to cope with her death, but I was still struggling with the idea of what to do with all of this information I had gained. How could I turn off the research switch in my brain when I still had this thirst for knowledge on the topic of cancer fighting foods and cancer prevention for my current and future pets? It was a part of my life now and it didn't seem logical to let this information go to waste.

This experience and Nola's disease meant more than that and I felt compelled to write it all down in a format I could reference later if, God forbid, I ever needed it again. The thought of going through all of the research again would not only be stupid, but daunting. I already put in the time and now I want to help others with the information I have learned *and* I don't want to forget any of it as well. That's how the idea for this book transpired. It was and is the only thing that gives me hope that all of this must have happened for a reason and her journey had a purpose.

Who knows, maybe I will end up with cancer some day and I will be thankful to have my reference book and the power of knowledge to fight the cancer head on. Or, maybe I was meant to help others fight it through Nola's experience. I don't know the reason, but I know that nothing happens without a purpose and I feel helping others through this experience, by sharing what we learned, will give Nola's journey the purpose and meaning it was always meant to have.

So, you guessed it, creating this book started out as therapy for me to fill the empty space of time, but it also helped me to make sense of it all. I'm not saying you have to write a book, but I would write something. Write down your feelings. Write about things you learned on your journey that you don't want to forget. Write a blog or a journal - just write it all down. You will be amazed how powerful it can be. Don't worry about writing well. I've never considered myself a strong writer and you may agree after reading this. I used to hate writing, before I had something to say. Now I get consumed with these urges to get it all down on paper that I can't control or explain. It has been an amazing release and it makes it possible for me to talk about Nola, without breaking down into tears, so that counts for something, right?

My last piece of advice for filling the empty space of time is to fill it with another pet if you don't already have another one, or even if you do. You need time to heal first, but once you are over the hump, don't feel guilty for wanting another animal. You have so much love to give, whether you are rescuing a senior or getting a new puppy or kitten, and you need to share that love with other animals because they need you too. We already had Barley, but I had always planned to get him another brother or sister sooner than later. Barley has some issues with insecurity and I didn't want him to remain an only child for too long. I felt the longer we waited the harder it would be for him to adjust back to the idea of sharing his space. I did not, however, expect to get a new dog within a month of Nola's passing, almost to the day, but that's what happened.

Even though I had started to see the light again, I felt it was too soon. I felt guilty for replacing my girl, but our new little girl, Suri, was found by a friend in the middle of a busy highway and needed a permanent home, or she was on her way to the local shelter. My heart couldn't let that happen, so I agreed to take her in, at least until we could find her a permanent home. Deep down, I knew that I would not part with her

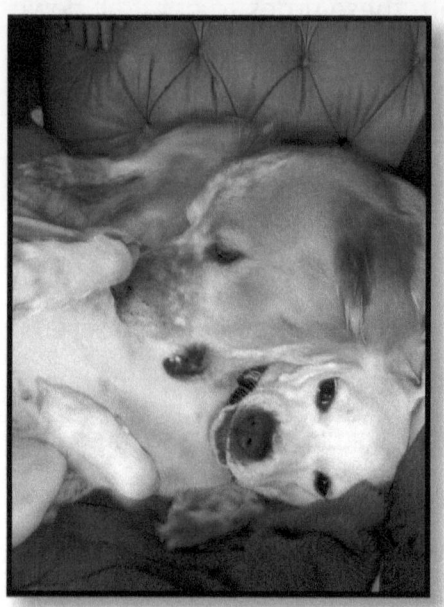

once I had her, but telling myself it was temporary was how I rationalized bringing her home. Barley and Suri became buddies almost immediately and she proved to be the perfect medicine for all of us. This picture of Suri and Barley was taken very soon after we found Suri and gave her a home. One would think they had been living together for years. I believe she saved Barley's heart as much as she did ours. Barley was missing his big sister and we all needed the distraction. All of a sudden, the rest of the empty space of time was filled with training a new puppy and watching Barley and Suri run around the yard. He had not had the opportunity to do this in a long time with another dog. Nola would get out and play a little, but only in short durations.

I know some of you will roll your eyes at this next statement, but I truly believe either God, Nola or my dad (or all three) played a part in bringing Suri into our lives at the perfect moment. She even looks like a small version of Nola, which for us was okay because she has a completely different personality. There was something about having that little white face in the house again that shined a bright light upon us and healed our home. That is why we named her Suri, which is short for Suriel, who is one of the angels who greets you into heaven when you pass. I believe Suri was heaven sent – someone knew my heart needed saving and I've been blessed all over again.

To conclude, I want to send you a virtual hug and tell you I am praying for each and every one of you who is on this journey with your awesome little badass cancer warrior. I pray if your warrior doesn't make it, you find ways to honor it, but that you also find time to heal. Cry it out and take care of your mental and physical health. Put its dog tag on your keychain, necklace or just keep it in your pocket, so that you can feel close to it again. Write down your thoughts and feelings. And, when you are ready, pour all of that love you have to give into a new little animal that needs a home. You can heal each other...it's powerful and it works.

I am so sorry you had to take this journey with us, but I hope our story and this book have empowered you along the way.

Godspeed cancer warriors.
Be brave. Be strong. Be in the moment.

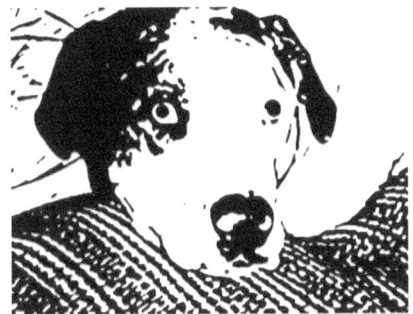

Appendix

Included within the appendix:

- ➤ Nola's Food /Supplement Chart
- ➤ Documents from Reggie Black (Better Way Health) about Beta 1 3D Glucan
- ➤ Information about Avemar (Shield4Pets)
- ➤ Yin & Yang Food Charts

Nola's Food / Supplement Chart

Item	12:00am	6:00am	9:00am	12:00pm	4:00pm	8pm
Artemis / Avemar / Essiac / Burdock / Slippery Elm						
Butyrex						
Budwigs w/ Greens						
Steel cut oats / Quinoa						
Flax Oil / Fish Oil						
Raw Honey / Bee Pollen						
Mushrooms / Beans / sweet potato						
Astragalus / Dandelion						
garlic & ginger						
NuVet / D3 / C / E / Potass +						
ACV H2O / lemon H2O						
Kefir / Egg Shells / cottage cheese						
Snack						
Plain Chicken						
Coconut Oil, Milk or Water						
Dried Grn Barley/ Wheat grass						
Bromelian / Bozwellia / White Willow / Curamed						
Tramadol / Piroxicam / Gabapentin						
Benedryl / Antibiotic						
BETA-1 Glucan / Vit C / Lysine / Proline / Grn T						
Vascu Statin						
Guaifenesin / Theophylline / Samshe Chuanbei Ye						

Documents from Reggie Black at Better Way Health about Beta1 3D Glucan

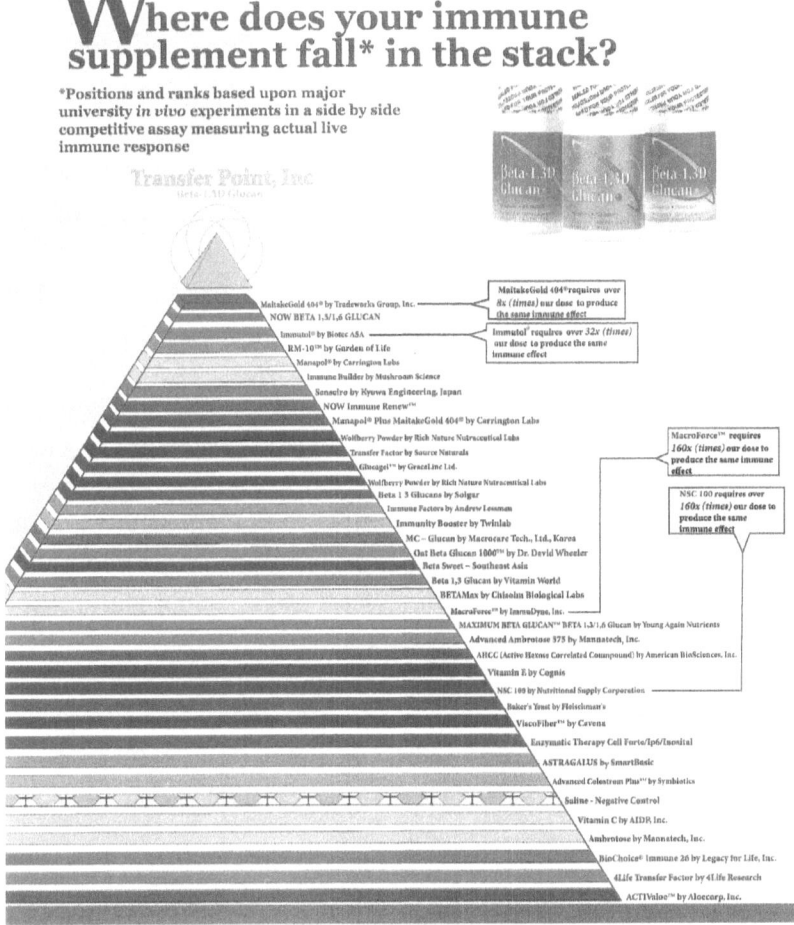

Where does your immune supplement fall* in the stack?

*Positions and ranks based upon major university *in vivo* experiments in a side by side competitive assay measuring actual live immune response

Transfer Point, Inc
Beta-1,3D Glucan

MaitakeGold 404® by Tradeworks Group, Inc.
NOW BETA 1,3/1,6 GLUCAN
Immutol® by Biotec ASA
RM-10™ by Garden of Life
Manapol® by Carrington Labs
Immune Builder by Mushroom Science
Sonastre by Kyowa Engineering, Japan
NOW Immune Renew™
Manapol® Plus MaitakeGold 404® by Carrington Labs
Wolfberry Powder by Rich Nature Nutraceutical Labs
Transfer Factor by Source Naturals
Glucagel™ by GraceLinc Ltd.
Wolfberry Powder by Rich Nature Nutraceutical Labs
Beta 1 3 Glucans by Solgar
Immune Factors by Andrew Lessman
Immunity Booster by Twinlab
MC – Glucan by Macrocare Tech., Ltd., Korea
Oat Beta Glucan 1000™ by Dr. David Wheeler
Beta Sweet – Southeast Asia
Beta 1,3 Glucan by Vitamin World
BETAMax by Chisolm Biological Labs
MacroForce™ by ImmuDyne, Inc.
MAXIMUM BETA GLUCAN™ BETA 1,3/1,6 Glucan by Young Again Nutrients
Advanced Ambrotose 375 by Mannatech, Inc.
AHCC (Active Hexose Correlated Compound) by American BioSciences, Inc.
Vitamin E by Cognis
NSC 100 by Nutritional Supply Corporation
Baker's Yeast by Fleischman's
ViscoFiber™ by Cavena
Enzymatic Therapy Cell Forte/Ip6/Inositol
ASTRAGALUS by SmartBasic
Advanced Colostrum Plus™ by Synbiotics
Saline - Negative Control
Vitamin C by AIDP, Inc.
Ambrotose by Mannatech, Inc.
BioChoice® Immune 26 by Legacy for Life, Inc.
4Life Transfer Factor by 4Life Research
ACTIValoe™ by Aloecorp, Inc.

> MaitakeGold 404® requires over 8x *(times)* our dose to produce the same immune effect

> Immutol® requires over 32x *(times)* our dose to produce the same immune effect

> MacroForce™ requires 160x *(times)* our dose to produce the same immune effect

> NSC 100 requires over 160x *(times)* our dose to produce the same immune effect

Contact us for information

info@transferpoint.com
TRANSFER POINT
SUPPLEMENTS BACKED BY SCIENTIFIC RESEARCH   Toll Free: 877-407-3999 Telephone: 803-561-0342 Fax: 803-561-9497 **www.transferpoint.com**

A Comparison of Injected and Orally Administered â-glucans

Vaclav Vetvicka, PhD*, Jana Vetvickova, MS
University of Louisville, Department of Pathology, Louisville, Kentucky

ABSTRACT

â-glucans have been extensively studied for their pharmacological effects. Despite in-depth research, little is known about the optimal dose and/or optimal route of application. In this paper, we are reporting the result of comparing the immunostimulating activities of four commercially available glucans differing both in their solubility and source. In addition, we compared intraperitoneal and oral application, and the differences between a single versus repeated doses.

Our data showed strong differences in activities of individual glucans, with glucan yeast-derived #300 being the best, and grain-derived ImmuneFiber being the worst. Furthermore, we demonstrated that oral delivery of glucan resulted in significant immunological activity, which albeit slightly lower, corresponded with injectable application. Depending on the applied dose, the effects of individual glucans were long-lasting and in some cases, lasted up to two weeks.

In conclusion, our report represents further evidence about differences among commercial glucans and shows that these biological response modifiers can be similarly active when used in both injectable and oral form.

Correspondence:
Vaclav Vetvicka, PhD
University of Louisville
Department of Pathology and Laboratory Medicine
511 S. Floyd, MDR Bldg., Rm. 224
Louisville, KY 40202
Phone: 502-852-1612 FAX: 502-852-1177
E-mail: vetvickavaclav@netscape.net

INTRODUCTION

Natural products, useful in treating or preventing various diseases, have been sought throughout the history of mankind. Most of these natural products are plagued with a common problem, i.e., the fact that they often represent a complex mixture of individual ingredients, each of which can contribute to their biological activities. Natural (1,3)-â-D-glucans from yeast, grain and mushrooms are well-established biological response modifiers,1,2 representing highly conserved structural components of cell walls in yeast, fungi, seaweed, or grain seeds.

Numerous types of glucans have been isolated from almost every species of yeast, grain and fungi. (1,3)- â-Dglucans have been extensively studied for their immunological and pharmacological effects. More than 2,000 papers describing the biological activities of glucans exist in the literature.3 Another advantage of glucans is the fact that all sufficiently purified polysaccharidic immunomodulators distinguish themselves by very low toxicity (*e.g.*, for mouse lentinan has LD50 > 1600 mg/kg4).

Despite detailed knowledge of the activities of many glucans, limited information is available regarding the mechanisms of action by orally delivered glucans. For some time, there were even suggestions that orally administered glucans have no activity at all. Only recently has more information about the mechanisms of action of orally delivered glucans become available.5,6

The limited number of papers dealing with the problems of glucan transfer through the gastrointestinal tract mainly focus on the fact that fluorescent-labeled glucan can be detected in cells isolated from various tissues.7 The studies of Ross's group indicated that orally-administered (1,3)- â-D-glucan is taken up by gastrointestinal macrophages and subsequently shuttled to the reticuloendothelial system and bone marrow. Recent observation found that both insoluble glucans and soluble seaweed-derived Phycarine have similarly pronounced effects when applied via intraperitoneal or oral administration.7,8,9

The aims of the present study were to follow up our previously published comparison of commercial â-glucans10 and to test the effect of different commercially available glucans on both the cellular and humoral branches of immune reactions using different routes of administration.

MATERIAL AND METHODS
Animals
Female, 6 to 10 week old BALB/c mice were purchased from the Jackson Laboratory (Bar Harbor, ME). All animal work was done according to the University of Louisville IACUC protocol. Animals were sacrificed by CO_2 asphyxiation.

Materials
RPMI 1640 medium, sodium citrate, dextran, ovalbumin, Ficoll-Hypaque, antibiotics, sodium azide, bovine serum albumin, Wright stain, Limulus lysate test E-TOXATE, Freund's adjuvant and Concanavalin A were obtained from Sigma Chemical Co. (St. Louis, MO). Fetal calf serum (FCS) was from Hyclone Laboratories (Logan, UT).â **-1,3 glucans** The glucans used in this study were purchased from the following companies: NOW BETA glucan from NOW FOODS (Bloomingdale, IL), Krestin from Biotec (Kureha Chemical Industries, Tokyo, Japan), Glucan #300 from Transfer Point (Columbia, SC), and ImmunoFiber from (Whole Control, Arvada, CO).

Glucan treatment
Individual glucans were applied either intraperitoneally or orally. The samples were collected at different intervals after either single or three ip. injections (100 mg of glucan/mouse) or after one day or a fourteen-day feeding with glucan-containing diet. All diets (Laboratory Rodent Diet 5001 enhanced with various doses of glucan) were formulated and prepared by Purina (Richmond, IN). Diet ingredients for all groups were identical except for the proportion of glucan.

Antibodies
For fluorescence staining, the following antibodies have been employed: anti-mouse CD4, CD8 and CD19, conjugated with FITC, which were purchased from Biosource (Camarillo, CA).

Flow cytometry
Cells were stained with monoclonal antibodies on ice in 12 x 75-mm glass tubes using standard techniques. Pellets of $5x10^5$ cells were incubated with 10 μl of FITClabeled antibodies (1 to 20 μg/ml in PBS) for 30 minutes on ice. After washing with cold PBS, the cells were re-suspended in PBS containing 1% BSA and 10 mM sodium azide. Flow cytometry was performed with a FACScan (Becton Dickinson, San Jose, CA) flow cytometer and the data from over 10,000 cells/samples were analyzed.

Phagocytosis
The technique that employs phagocytosis of synthetic polymeric microspheres was described earlier.[11,12] Briefly: peritoneal cells were incubated with 0.05 ml of 2-hydroxyethyl methacrylate particles (HEMA; $5x10^8$/ml). The test tubes were incubated at 37° C for 60 min., with intermittent shaking. Smears were stained with Wright stain. The cells with three or more HEMA particles were considered positive. The same smears were also used for evaluation of cell types.

Evaluation of IL-2 production
Purified spleen cells ($2x10^6$/ml in RPMI 1640 medium with 5% FCS) were added into wells of a 24-well tissue culture plate. After the addition of 1 mg of Concanavalin A into positive-control wells, cells were incubated for 72 hrs. in a humidified incubator (37°C, 5% CO_2). At the endpoint of incubation, supernatants were collected, filtered through 0.45 mm filters and tested for the presence of IL-2. Levels of the IL-2 were measured using a Quantikine mouse IL-2 kit (R&D Systems, Minneapolis, MN).

RESULTS

Most published studies describe effects of injected â- glucans (either ip., iv. or sc.). However, it is necessary, in the event of clinical practice, to evaluate the possibility of oral delivery. Phagocytosis is one of the biological activities traditionally connected with effects of immunomodulators, including glucans. Therefore, we started our study by comparing the effects of orally and intraperitoneally applied glucans. When used as a single dose, ip. application showed more profound effects than oral application (Figure 1 A,B). In addition, some glucans (such as NOW and Krestin) exhibited either longer effects or were effective only after injection. When we repeated the glucan administration for three consecutive days, we found not only higher phagocytic activity, but that it also lasted significantly longer (in the case of #300 and Krestin, up to 7 days). Oral delivery also showed higher effects, but similar to a single dose, significant effects were observed only in the case of #300 (Figure 2 A,B). Next, we evaluated the effects of our glucans on the expression of some immunologically important surface markers on spleen lymphocytes isolated from mice stimulated with individual glucans. Using ip. injection, we found that 24 hrs. later, all glucans increased expression of CD4, but this effect was long-lasting only in the case of #300 (Figure 3A). When testing CD8 expression, the effects of three active glucans, #300, NOW and Krestin, were observed for 48 hrs. (Figure 4 A). None of the tested glucans affected the number of CD19-positive cells (B lymphocytes (Figure 5A). A similar situation has been found in orally-stimulated mice; the only exception was no activity of ImmunoFiber (Figures 3B,4B). Again, no effects on expression of CD19 (Figure 5B).

Production of IL-2 belongs to the valuable indicators of the immune activities. Therefore, we compared the effects of tested glucans on the secretion of IL-2 by spleen cells isolated from glucan-treated mice. The IL-2 production was measured after a 72 hr. *in vitro* incubation of cells. The results, summarized in Figure 6, showed that even when all tested glucan stimulated IL-2 production, there were huge differences between individual glucans (i.e., #300 stimulated IL-2 secretion 3.5 times more than ImmunoFiber). The activity of all tested glucans slowly decreased with time, but was still measurable 14 days after injection (Figure 6A). Virtually identical, albeit lower, results were found in the case of orally-treated mice (Figure 6B). When we evaluated the IL-2 production after repeated stimulation with glucans, we found a higher overall secretion of IL-2. Using ip. injection, #300 was more active than Concanavalin A up to seven days after last application, with both Krestin and NOW showing strong stimulation (Figure 7A). The same situation was found after oral application, where we discovered significant stimulation in each glucan even two weeks after the last application (Figure 7B). It is important to note that the secretion of IL-2 by control (i.e., non-stimulated cells) was almost zero; therefore, all glucans yielded statistically significant stimulations. When compared to stimulation with Con A, #300 showed stronger effects, Krestin and NOW were comparable, and ImmunoFiber showed lower activity.

Glucans are usually considered more as stimulators of the cellular branch of immune reactions; however, some glucans can act as nonspecific adjuvant. Using an experimental model of ovalbumin immunization, we applied glucan either intraperitoneally together with two doses of antigen (Figure 8A), or orally for two weeks (Figure 8B). In both cases, only glucans #300, Krestin and ImmunoFiber showed stimulation of antibody response. Finally, we evaluated whether the glucan feeding was reflected in changes of weight of individual organs. As seen in Table 1, there were no differences in the weight of any tested organs. In addition, the ip. injection had no effects (results not shown).

DISCUSSION

â-Glucans show notable physiological effects, which is the main reason why so much attention has been devoted to them. They belong to a group of physiologically active compounds, collectively termed biological response modifiers. Thus far, among many known and tested immunomodulators of the first order, polysaccharides isolated from different microorganisms and plants hold a formidable place.

A large number of such polysaccharides, that act only as immunopotentiators are well known.13 Binding of â-glucan to specific receptors (either CR3 or Dectin-1) activates macrophages. The activation consists of several interconnected processes including increased chemokinesis, chemotaxis, migration of macrophages, degranulation leading to increased expression of adhesive molecules, and adhesion to the endothelium. In addition, â- glucan binding triggers intracellular processes, characterized by the respiratory burst after phagocytosis of invading cells (formation of reactive oxygen species and free radicals), the increase of content and activity of hydrolytic enzymes, and signaling processes leading to activation of other cells and secretion of cytokines. For an excellent review regarding interaction of glucans with macrophages, see Schepetkin and Quinn.14

Regarding the question as to whether glucans are similarly active when administered orally, we compared the oral and intraperitoneal applications. To allow our experiments more relevancy in the use of natural immunostimulants, we compared the effects of a single application with repeated doses.

The rationale for the choice of glucans parallels what was stated in our previous paper.10 We chose four glucans widely sold and available in the US, Europe, and the Far East, representing grain-, mushroom- and yeast-derived glucans in soluble and insoluble form. Briefly, #300 is insoluble yeast-derived glucan; Krestin is soluble mushroom derived glucan; ImmunoFiber represents soluble grainderived glucan; and NOW is a mixture of both insoluble glucans from yeast and soluble glucans from mushrooms.

There are very few comprehensive reviews focused on biological properties of glucans from various existing sources. The comparative reviews focus mainly on the reflection of chemical characteristics of glucans on their biological and immunological properties.15,16

In this paper, we continued the comparison of several commercially important glucans.10 Glucans are well known for their ability to stimulate the innate immunity and the cellular branch of immune reaction.13 Therefore, our initial focus was phagocytic activity with the use of peripheral blood neutrophils and synthetic microspheres as a model. Our results confirmed our previous studies showing that glucan #300 was one of the most active glucans, regardless of the route of application.8,10,17-19 Additional data showed that the duration of these effects depends on the strength and timing of the glucan treatment since repeated doses clearly resulted in stronger and longer action stimulation. We then turned our attention to the effect of glucans on surface markers. In the case of CD4-positive lymphocytes, one injection of any of the glucans was enough to increase the influx of these cells. In the case of oral application, the data were similar with the exception of ImmunoFiber, which showed no activity. Similar data were observed in the case of CD8-positive splenocytes. In both cases, only #300, Krestin and NOW showed longer effects — two days for Krestin and NOW, and up to one week for glucan #300. The number of CD19-positive cells (B lymphocytes) did not change. These findings were in agreement with previous data established using Phycarine20 or lentinan.21 When we measured repeated doses of glucan, the results were identical to those shown in Figures 3 to 5, and due to the restricted space, were not included in this report.

It is assumed that glucan application results in signaling processes leading to activation of macrophages and other cells, and subsequent secretion of cytokines and other substances initiating inflammation reactions (*e.g.*, interleukins IL-1, IL-2, IL-6, and TNF-á).22-24

We found that all tested glucans stimulated splenocytes to produce IL-2, with #300 and Krestin showing the strongest and longest effects. Our findings were similar to previously published data.8,10,20

As some recent studies established that glucans can also support the humoral branch of the immune reaction by serving as adjuvant,25 we compared the adjuvant activities of tested glucans with Freund's adjuvant. Our results showed that even when the activities were always lower than those of Freund's adjuvant, they were nevertheless significant, with the higher activity found in the previously almost inactive ImmunoFiber. These data correlate well with the previous finding of significant adjuvant activity with grainderived glucans.10 It is important to note that in these experiments, we applied the glucans either two times ip. (together with the antigen) or for a full two weeks (in case of oral application).

The present paper represents yet another proof of vast differences among commercially available glucans. To conclude — glucan #300 was again a highly active glucan with a sufficiently broad range of action. We demonstrated that oral application is comparable to the intraperitoneal route, and that the somehow lower effects after oral stimulation can be easily overcome by repeated oral doses.

ACKNOWLEDGEMENT

The authors thank Ms. Rosemary Williams for excellent editorial assistance.

DISCLAIMER

The authors of this study have no significant financial interest in any of the products or manufacturers mentioned in the article. No external funding was provided for this study.

REFERENCES

1. Borchers AT, Stern JS, Hackman RM, Keen CL, Gershwin ME. Mushrooms, tumors, and immunity. *Proc Soc Exp Biol Med.* 1999; 221:281-293.
2. Brown GD, Gordon S. Fungal b-glucans and mammalian immunity. *Immunity.* 2003; 19:311-315.
3. Novak M, Vetvicka V. Beta-glucans, history and present. *Alt Med Rev* 2007, in press.

4. Chihara G, Maeda YY, Hamuro J. Current status and perspectives of immunomodulators of microbial origin. *Int J Tis React.* 1982; IV:207-225.

5. Hong F, Yan J, Baran JT, Allendorf DJ, Hansen RD, Ostroff GR, Xing PX, Cheung NK, Ross GD. Mechanism by which orally administered b-1,3-glucans enhance the tumoricidal activity of antitumor monoclonal antibodies in murine tumor models. *J Immunol.* 2004; 173:797-806.

6. Vetvicka V, Dvorak B, Vetvickova J, Richter J, Krizan J, Sima P, Yvin JC. Orally administered marine (1->3)- b-D-glucan Phycarine stimulates both humoral and cellular immunity. *Int J Biol Macromol.* 2006; 40:291-298.

7. Li B, Allendorf DJ, Hansen R, Marroquin J, Ding C, Cramer DE, Yan J. Yeast b-glucan amplifies phagocyte killing of iC3b-opsonized tumor cells via complement receptor 3-Syk-Phosphatidylinositol 3-kinase pathway. *J Immunol.* 2006; 177:1661-1669.

8. Allendorf DJ, Baran JT, Hansen RD, Subbarao K, Walsh D, Hong F, Marroquin J, Yan J. Orally administered bglucan functions via anti-tumor mAbs and the complement system to recruit CR3+ neutrophils and JANA Vol. 11, No. 1, 2008 49 macrophages that produce tumor regression and tumorfree survival. *Mol Immunol.* 2003; 40:195-196.

9. Yan J, Allendorf DJ, Brandley B. Yeast whole glucan particle (WGP) beta-glucan in conjunction with antitumor monoclonal antibodies to treat cancer. *Expert Opin Biol Ther.* 2005; 5:691-702.

10. Vetvicka V, Vetvickova J. An evaluation of the immunological activities of commercially available b1,3-glucans. *JANA.* 2007; 10:25-31.

11. Vetvicka V, Fornusek L, Kopecek J, Kaminkova J, Kasparek L, Vranova M. Phagocytosis of human blood leukocytes: a simple micromethod. *Immunol Lett.* 1982; 5:97-100.

12. Vetvicka V, Holub M, Kováru H, Siman P, Kováru F. Alpha-fetoprotein and phagocytosis in athymic nude mice. *Immunol Lett.* 1988; 19:95-98.

13. Whistler RL, Bushway AA, Singh PP, Nakahara W, Tokuzen R. Noncytotoxic, antitumor polysaccharides. *Adv Carbohydr Chem Biochem.* 1976; 32:235-275.

14. Schepetkin IA, Quinn MT. Botanical polysaccharides: macrophage immunomodulation and therapeutical potential. *Int Immunopharmacol.* 2006; 6:317-333.

15. Yadomae T. Structure and biological activities of fungal b-1,3-glucans. *Yakugaku Zasshi.*2000; 120:413-431.

16. Kogan G. (1-3,1-6)-b-D-glucans of yeast and fungi and their biological activity. In: Atta-ur-Rahman, (ed): Studies in Natural Products Chemistry. Amsterdam, *Elsevier.* 2000: 107-152.

17. Kurashige S, Akuzawa Y, Endo F. Effects of Lentinus edodes, Grifola frondosa and Pleurotus ostreatus administration on cancer outbreak, and activities of macrophages and lymphocytes in mice treated with a carcinogen, Nbutyl- N-butanolnitrosoamine. *Immunopharmacol Immunotoxicol.* 1997;19:175-183.

18. Vetvicka V, Vetvicka J. Physiological effects of different types of â-glucan. Biomed. Pap. 2007;151:1-7.

19. Vetvicka V, Vetvickova J. Immunostimulating properties of two different b-glucans isolated from Maitake mushrooms (*Grifola frondosa*). *JANA.* 2005; 8:33-39. 20. Vetvicka V, Yvin JC. Effects of marine beta-1,3 glucan on immune reactions. *Int Immunopharmacol.* 2004; 4:721-730.

21. Arinaga S, Karimine N, Takamuku K, Nanbara S, Nagamatsu M, Ueo H, Akiyoshi T. Enhanced production of interleukin 1 and tumor necrosis factor by peripheral monocytes after lentinan administration in patients with gastric carcinoma. *Int J Immunopharmacol.* 1992; 14:43-47.

22. Adachi Y, Okazaki M, Ohno N, Yadomae T. Enhancement of cytokine production by macrophages stimulated with (1->3)- b-D-glucan, Grifolan (GRN), isolated from *Grifola frondosa*. *Biol Pharm Bull.* 1994; 17:1554-1560.

23. Abel G, Czop JK. Stimulation of human monocyte bglucan receptors by glucan particles induces production of TNF-a and IL-1b. *Int J Immunopharmacol.* 1992; 14:1363-1373.

24. Vetvicka V, Terayama K, Mandeville R, Brousseau P, Kournikakis B, Ostroff G. Pilot study: orally administered yeast b1,3-glucan

prophylactically protects against anthrax infection and cancer in mice. *JANA*. 2002; 5:1-6.

25. Cook JA, Holbrook TW. Immunogenicity of soluble and particulate antigens from *Leishmania donovani:* effect of glucan as an adjuvant. *Infect Immun*. 1984; 40:1038-1043.

The research is clear and trillions of white blood cells agree that Transfer Point's Glucan #300 tops them all.

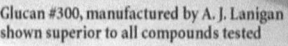

Glucan #300, manufactured by A. J. Lanigan shown superior to all compounds tested

Compounds requiring over 8x the dose of Glucan #300 for same immune effect
• PSK Krestin by Kureha Corp.
• MaitakeGold 404® by Tradeworks Group, Inc.
• Beta 1,3/1,6 Glucan by NOW®

Compounds requiring over 32x the dose of Glucan #300 for same immune effect
• Epicor™ by Diamond V
• Immutol® by Biotec ASA
• RM-10™ by Garden of Life

Compounds requiring over 64x the dose of Glucan #300 for same immune effect
• BioBran® by Daiwa Pharmaceutical Co., Ltd.
• Manapol® by Carrington Labs
• Immune Builder® by Mushroom Science
• Senseiro by Kyowa Engineering, Japan
• Immune Renew™ by NOW®
• Manapol® Plus MaitakeGold 404® by Carrington Labs
• Wolfberry Powder by Rich Nature™ Nutraceutical Labs
• Transfer Factor™ by Source Naturals®
• Glucagel™ by GraceLinc Ltd.
• Beta Glucan 1,3 Glucans by Solgar®
• Immune Factors™ by Andrew Lessman
• Immunity Booster™ by Twinlab®
• MC-Glucan by Macrocare Tech., Ltd., Korea
• Oat Beta Glucan 1000™ by Dr. David Wheeler
• Beta Sweet-Southeast Asia
• Beta 1,3 Glucan by Vitamin World
• BETAMax by Chisolm Biological Labs

Compounds requiring over 160x the dose of Glucan #300 for same immune effect
• MacroForce™ by ImmuDyne, Inc.
• Maximum Beta Glucan™ by Young Again Nutrients
• Advanced Ambrotose™ 375 by Mannatech, Inc.
• AHCC ImmPOWER™ (Active Hexose Correlated Compound) by American BioSciences, Inc.
• Vitamin C by Cognis
• NSC 100™ by Nutritional Supply Corporation
• Baker's Yeast by Fleischman's®
• ViscoFiber™ by Cevena
• Cell Forte/IP6/Inositol by Enzymatic Therapy
• ASTRAGALUS by SmartBasic
• Advanced Colostrom Plus™ by Symbiotics

These products produced less effect than saline, the negative control
• Vitamin C by AIDP, Inc.
• Ambrotose by Mannatech, Inc.
• BioChoice® Immune 26 by Legacy for Life, Inc.
• 4Life® Transfer Factor™ by 4Life Research
• ACTIValoe™ by Aloecorp, Inc.

IF you are looking for an immune support supplement, now is the time to discover Transfer Point's Beta glucan. Continuously and thoroughly tested for safety and efficacy by leading universities and teaching hospitals.

The supplements listed at left all claim to benefit the immune system. Each was third party tested and not one single supplement evaluated was close to matching the immune enhancing capabilities of our Beta glucan.

We don't just claim Transfer Point's Beta glucan can enhance the immune response, we prove it.

"Glucan #300 showed a broad range of action. Glucan #300 was the biologically most relevant immunomodulator."
–Dr. Vaclav Vetvicka, PhD, University of Louisville

"When I share Beta-1,3D Glucan with my patients, I know they have a safe and effective product that meets their healthcare needs."–Kalyani M. Kumar, M.D., F.A.C.O.G., President and Chief Medical Officer, American Wellness Alliance, Richmond, Virginia.

"After 30 years of dental surgery, I found a biological response modifier that I use along with the standard of care to help deal with antibiotic resistance, post operative complications, allergic reactions and other complex issues."
–John L. Tate, DDS, Spartanburg, SC

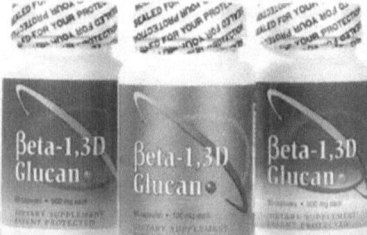

AVEMAR

Avemar is fermented wheat germ that has been put through many different processes to achieve its remarkable capabilities. It was discovered in Hungary where it is widely used but now is also gaining acceptance in the United States. Memorial Sloan Kettering Cancer Institute has been recognizing the value of this product in treating cancer patients. I'll try to explain how it works but it works in many different ways, on a cellular level to destroy cancer cells or at the least, to remove their ability to thrive.

The mutated genes in cancer cells constantly urge these malignant cells to divide. In order to maintain the processes of cell division, cell metabolism must also be changed; the cell needs to adapt nucleic acids (RNA/DNA) and other constituents. Cancer cells adapt their metabolism, to gain energy, in a way that enables them to utilize the most abundant resource in circulation: *glucose*. (This is why so many "cancer diets" are based on no carbohydrates and no sugars.). In order to maintain a continuous proliferation, it is crucial that glucose is utilized continuously for synthetic (anabolic) biochemical processes.

Tumor cells can and do easily adapt to a glucose-based metabolism; they are capable of taking up enormous quantities of this molecule - up to *20-30 times more than normal cells.* One part of this glucose is used by cancer cells for energy production, while another part will be used for the synthesis of nucleic acids, which are the building blocks of RNA and DNA.

To make a very complex group of processes simple for us lay people, the way Avemar works is to decrease the glucose-uptake of tumor cells in a dose-dependent manner and inhibits the production of ribose and deoxyribose, a sugar that is the backbone of DNA. It also inhibits key enzymes that cancer cells need to grow. Further, Avemar enhances TNFalpha (tumor necrosis factor alpha) production, thereby inhibiting tumor angiogenesis. Angiogenesis is the ability of cancer cells to keep itself well supplied with blood. It produces an enzyme that tells the circulatory system to send up more circulation or blood supply. Think of it as an evil entity that circumvents the natural processes in the body to establish an evil empire which builds itself into a monster! Avemar deconstructs cancer cells by working in many of these processes, turning them back into what they were before the onslaught of cancer which took control and cleverly used these natural processes to grow at an enormous rate.

Avemar also has an immune modulating effect by exerting a selective inhibition of MHC-I (main histocompatibility-I) expression on the surface of tumor cells. Avemar seems to restore the immune system to its pre-damaged condition. The MHC genes are responsible for regulating antibody recognition which means Avemar is useful in autoimmune diseases, as well.

There have been hundreds of clinical studies with Avemar throughout the world and in the United States. Many of these studies showed that Avemar induces apoptosis or programmed cell death of cancer cells after the first 24 hours of use. It also has significant anti-inflammatory effects and supports detoxification, aiding the body in disposing of the dead cancer cells and any toxins formed in the process of apoptosis.

It is used in conjunction with all forms of chemotherapy and has been proven to extend survival time and quality of life in human patients without any side effects except a loose stool. It should not be taken at the same time as vitamin C. Otherwise there are no restrictions. It is taken on an empty stomach 2 hours after any other food or supplement and 2 hours before feeding. It comes in a packet but I put it into capsules since my dog will not touch it as an addition to her food. I have a very finicky eater! I used frozen yogurt to mix with her capsules and yogurt is one of the allowable ways to administer Avemar.

Jazzie died on October 4, 2008, not from the cancer but from lysing. She died as she was removed from the x-ray table—cardiac failure but the x-rays gave us some hint about how well

Avemar worked. There were none of the classical signs of lung mets—instead, she had fluid build-up from lysing which is the result of tumors being destroyed. The dangers of treating lung tumors is the possibility of these secretions. I don't think I could have done anything differently because Jazzie had a very serious adverse reaction to Neoplasene and could not take it longer than 3 months. During that time, Neoplasene had completely arrested the growths. We had no choice but to use Avemar. If anything, Avemar worked too well.

I purchase Avemar at www.iherb.com

Barbara Bouyet

bouyet@roadrunner.com

Yin & Yang Food Charts

Yin Acid-forming foods

Sugar, sweeteners
Oils
Nuts
Beans
Pasta, Flour
Vinegar, Alcoholic Beverages
(Also: drugs, pills)

Yin Alkaline-forming foods

Fruit juice, Herb teas, Bancha tea,
Coffee (organic, w/caffeine)
Water
Cocoa (unsweetened, Dutch treated)
Fruit
Seeds
Vegetables
Honey, Spices

Yang Acid-forming foods

Grains — (except Millet)
Animal Foods — (Fish,
Poultry, Beef, Pork,
Eggs,
Salted Cheese, etc.)

Yang Alkaline-forming foods

Millet
Wakame & Kombu Seaweeds
Lotus, Burdock, & Dandelion roots
Jinenjo (Japanese potato)
Salt (unrefined sea salt)
Gomashio (sesame salt)
Soy sauce, Miso , Umeboshi plum
Kuzu, Dandelion, & Mu teas,
Yannoh (Ohsawa coffee)
Ginseng

The Balance Chart

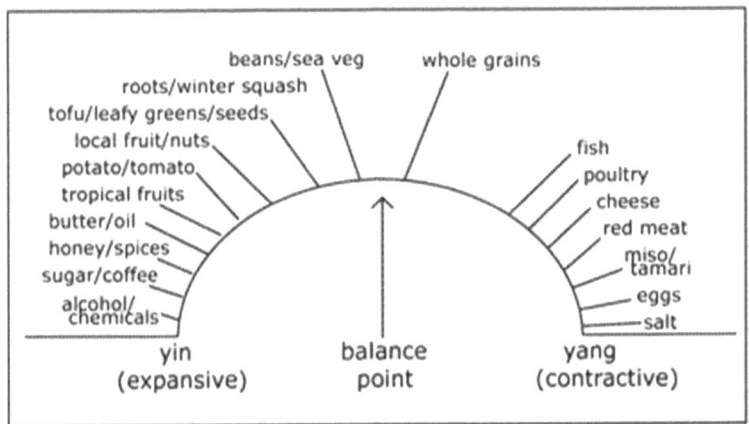

beans/sea veg
roots/winter squash
tofu/leafy greens/seeds
local fruit/nuts
potato/tomato
tropical fruits
butter/oil
honey/spices
sugar/coffee
alcohol/chemicals

whole grains

fish
poultry
cheese
red meat
miso/tamari
eggs
salt

yin
(expansive)

balance
point

yang
(contractive)

About Heather

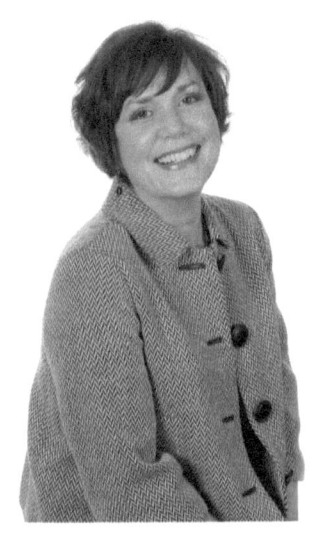 Heather Beuke Diers is an artist with many areas of expertise – interior design, original art and custom furniture. Recently she has added published author and blogger to her artistic montage by writing about her true passions in life, animals and holistic healthcare. Natural medicine is an artistic form of its own and Heather uses a palette of herbs, spices and essential oils to heal the body as well as the soul. She has spent years researching the best holistic cancer cures and preventions for both animals and humans.

Although Heather is an artist by trade, anyone who knows her personally thinks of her first as an animal lover and nutrition enthusiast. She understands animals benefit from proper nutrition and holistic care as much as we do and Mother Nature gives us everything we need to prevent most diseases. Heather's mission is to educate others on the importance of proper nutrition to heal the body.

You can follow Heather's blog at heathersholisticpawprints.com and her Facebook page, facebook.com/heathersholisticpawprints.com.

www.ingramcontent.com/pod-product-compliance
Lightning Source LLC
Chambersburg PA
CBHW030931180526
45163CB00002B/531